The Heart
of the Matter

♥

*Essential Advice for a Healthy Heart from
Renowned Surgeons and Cardiologists*

THIRD EDITION

HILTON M. HUDSON, II, M.D., F.A.C.S.

KAROL E. WATSON, M.D., PH.D., F.A.C.C.

RICHARD ALLEN WILLIAMS, M.D.

Hilton Publishing Company
Chicago, Illinois

© 2000, 2008 by Hilton Publishing Company

Hilton Publishing Company
Chicago, IL

Direct all correspondence to:
Hilton Publishing Company
1630 45th Street, Suite 103
Munster, IN 46321
219-922-4868
www.hiltonpub.com

ISBN: 0-9743144-4-7
ISBN 13: 978-09743144-4-0

Notice: The information in this book is true and complete to the best of the author's and publisher's knowledge. This book is intended only as an informative reference and should not replace, countermand, or conflict with the advice given to readers by their physicians. The authors and publisher disclaim all liability in connection with the specific personal use of any and all information provided in this book. References to real people, events, establishments, organizations, or locales are intended only to provide a sense of authenticity and are used fictitiously.

Library of Congress Cataloging-in-Publication Data

Heart of the matter : essential advice for a healthy heart from renowned surgeons and cardiologists / Hilton M. Hudson, II . . . [et al.].
    p. cm.
Originally published: 2000. ISBN 0-9743144-4-7
        1.Coronaryheartdisease.2.Hypertension.3.AfricanAmericans—Healthand hygiene. 4. African Americans—Diseases.
I. Hudson, Hilton M.

RC685.C6H785   2008
616.1'23--dc22   2007051956

Printed and bound in the United States of America
Distributed by SCB Distributors

Contents

Acknowledgments

DR. HILTON HUDSON'S ACKNOWLEDGMENTS

My sincere gratitude to my mentors and friends who continue to inspire me: Dr. George Rawls, Dr. P. David Myerowitz, Mr. Joe E. Robert, and my father, Rev. Hilton M. Hudson Sr.

DR. KAROL WATSON'S ACKNOWLEDGMENTS

The strength and support of my husband, Dr. Christopher Branche, has made all of my accomplishments possible. My beautiful children Afton, Logan, Kaycee and Corrie keep me focused on the goal of preventing unnecessary deaths from heart disease.

My greatest respect and thanks go to my parents and to all of my mentors, with special thanks to Drs. Judah Folkman, Alan Fogelman, and Gregg Fonarow. And lastly, I thank my patients who have taught me as much as I hope I have taught them, and who have contributed to this book with their remarkable courage, spirit, and strength.

Preface

THE CENTRAL MESSAGE OF THIS BOOK is that fear kills and courage saves lives. For many, preventing a heart attack or stroke equates to a kind of magical ritual—"If I just don't think about it, don't let it into my mind, I'll be safe from harm" or "If I sit still and hardly breathe, maybe serious physical harm and even death won't know that I am here."

Unfortunately, this type of thinking doesn't work or, more exactly, it works against us. Fear goes hand in hand with denial. Denial keeps us from visiting our doctors who can detect early warning signs like high cholesterol and high blood pressure. These warning signs can be detected at a stage where they can be treated by medication and by life style changes that give us longer and happier lives.

Having heart courage means transforming fear into positive action. The first part of that action is understanding your subject—how heart attacks and strokes happen, who they're most likely to happen to, how diet and exercise keep the heart strong, how to manage stress that might otherwise lead to threats to the heart, how heart surgery works, and what doctors can do, with our active help, to ensure that we recover from a heart attack if we experience one. We wrote this book with the conviction that people who have knowledge will find the courage to take their health into their own hands.

In *The Heart of the Matter* you will meet people like yourselves, wrestling with health situations and conditions just like those that you or people around you are wrestling with. Yes, coronary artery disease is the leading killer of Americans, and it hits African Americans harder than White Americans, Latino Americans, and any other community in the United States. But no one has to be a victim. Reading this book gives you the opportunity to learn from the experiences of others, and to understand how your heart works. And, you are being given a chance to work with your doctor to fix your heart when it doesn't work as it should.

Our highest hope is that you finish reading this book committed to keeping your own heart healthy. The key, after all, is *prevention*. And we know, from past experience, that people with the right kind of knowledge teach it to loved ones and friends. In that way, you not only learn how to make necessary changes for yourself, but you can also become an active participant in the battle against heart disease in which doctors and patients stand together.

The Heart
of the Matter

Chapter 1

Heart Courage

PEOPLE FEAR HEART ATTACKS for a variety of reasons. Some are afraid because family members or friends have been stricken, so heart attacks begin to feel too close to home. Others have already had one heart attack, and the fact that they were lucky to have survived—one in three victims of heart attacks die of them—makes them especially fearful. Fear can turn into panic and panic can kill. People can get so panicked by the possibility of a heart attack that when they actually have one they die unnecessarily.

Fear also goes hand in hand with denial. People do not go in for annual checkups because they fear that the doctor will find something wrong with their heart. They avoid knowing anything about the subject, as if by hiding behind a wall of ignorance they could protect themselves.

That is why I urge my patients and you to have "heart courage"—

Even people who have already had heart attacks can learn what they need to do in order to recover to full health and help prevent another attack from happening.

1

that is, do not live in fear of heart attacks or other heart malfunctions. Heart courage means turning fear into care and prevention. It means knowing what you need to do to give yourself the best protection against a heart attack. Even people who have already had heart attacks can learn what they need to do in order to recover to full health and to help prevent another attack from happening.

Facts are the best protection against panic, so here are some key facts:

1. You can help prevent a heart attack by taking care of yourself through proper diet, exercise, and avoidance of health risks such as smoking, physical inactivity, and unnecessary psychological stress.

2. Regular visits to the doctor will aid in detecting problems that may eventually damage the heart, such as the presence of high blood pressure, also known as hypertension.

3. If one of your parents or siblings has had a heart problem, there may be a family tendency toward heart trouble. Knowing of such history, your doctor may recommend a preventive program that lowers your own risk.

4. Educating yourself about health matters is a big step toward heart courage. You need to know how the body works and how illness occurs and should be treated.

5. One-and-a-half million heart attacks occur in the United States each year, and heart attacks are the #1 killer of Americans—higher than stroke, cancer, HIV/AIDS, or violence.

Many people know more about the way their car is made

and how it works than about their own bodies! Denial or lack of knowledge about how your heart works and how things can go wrong can make you vulnerable to accepting myths and incorrect information about your heart and can cause anxiety, which is basically a fear of the unknown.

Reading books like this is already a giant step towards educating yourself about your heart. True knowledge is the best preventive medicine and will help to fortify you with Heart Courage. Many pharmacies also supply free pamphlets on various health subjects, and you should avail yourself of material written by health professionals whom you can trust.

You can also get heart-health information from newspapers and magazines, and by visiting health fairs where screenings are done for high blood pressure, diabetes, and cholesterol levels. These fairs give you the opportunity to ask health professionals questions about your heart.

Of course, your ultimate source of information about your heart is your doctor, and you should always discuss any information that you have acquired on your own with a doctor.

What if you do everything you can to learn more about your heart and do all the right things to keep it healthy, and you have a heart attack anyway? How does the concept of Heart Courage help you then? Does it apply to a situation where your life is actually hanging in the balance? This is when you *most* need courage. Surviving a heart attack is a triumph in itself, because at least a third of all heart attack victims die with the first attack, and half of the remaining group die within a month.

So you are a survivor who now must focus on trying to prevent the next event, since heart attacks occur most frequently in people who have already had one. The plan you enter into with your doctor is called "secondary prevention," and it is like being given a second chance to avoid death. Taking hold of this opportunity requires that you gain the initiative, strength, will power, and sheer desire to go on living. Such determined planning is the essence of Heart Courage, and it is done in partnership with your doctor.

Your physician should help you to develop Heart Courage from the very moment that you are stabilized in the hospital. The doctor should not only console and comfort you but should also assure you that you are going to be all right and that you need to start to work right away on rehabilitating yourself.

Your doctor's guidance begins in the hospital with the doctor explaining what happened to your heart. He or she should also explain that a heart attack is not the end of the world and that, with good medical guidance, you are going to begin to repair what can be repaired and adjust to whatever permanent damage was done. Finally, your doctor should outline a plan for progressive rehabilitation. In the beginning, you may need rehabilitation to help you recover your strength.

While you are still in the hospital you will want to ask the doctor such questions as:

- Why did this happen to me?
- Will it happen again?
- How will this affect my ability to lead a normal life, enjoy living, and engage in satisfying activities, including sexual activity?
- What precautions must I take in doing these things?
- What can I eat, and what should I avoid?

Let's look at Renée Martin—a 50-year-old African-American female who lives with her husband and three children in Miami, Florida. She has been employed for ten years as a travel agent with a large company. Her husband is employed as a realtor, and together they make enough money to own a home, pay for private schooling for their children, and have an occasional dinner out at a nice restaurant. They have saved for their children's college education but they have concerns about the escalating costs of college. Renée would like to earn more money but she has been frustrated in her attempts to find a higher-paying job. She has been under a great deal of stress because of these financial concerns.

Renée's doctor recently made the diagnosis of high blood pressure and told her that she must lose 20 pounds of weight and get involved in an exercise program. She has been taking a "water pill" for the high blood pressure but this medicine has not controlled it. Although she joined a gym, she has difficulty attending more than once or twice a week because of her work schedule and duties at home, and many weeks she does not attend at all.

Renée's mother had a heart attack at age 52, and at 72 years of age she has a very limited life. Renée's father died of a stroke at 65 years of age after having had uncontrolled high blood pressure for years. A maternal aunt and a sister have adult-onset diabetes.

In the past month, Renée started experiencing occasional discomfort in her chest just beneath the breastbone. It does not go to other parts of her body, and it sometimes is and sometimes is not associated with activity. It lasts for just a few seconds. Renée thought it might be indigestion or "gas pains," so she tried antacids, but they did not work.

When Renée talked to her mother about it, her mother said that this was the way that her own heart attack had started, with months of strange chest pains gradually becoming more severe and lasting longer. The pains even awakened her from sleep. After that conversation, Renée felt doomed to repeat the scenario that her mother had experienced. She feared for her life.

At this point, what do you think Renée should do? Should she try some other over-the-counter medicines? What about eating less "gassy" food and cutting out things like ham, barbeque, and meatballs? Should she buy some herbal supplements and vitamins? Maybe she should cut down on coffee and substitute green tea. Will prayer help?

Actually, the first thing she should do is to consult her doctor and tell him about these new symptoms. This should prompt the doctor to investigate things more completely by taking a new and more thorough history, doing a complete physical examination, and ordering some special tests including an electrocardiogram (EKG), a chest x-ray, and a series of blood tests. He may refer Renée to a cardiologist for an expert opinion about whether she has coronary artery disease (CAD).

After making the diagnosis of CAD, he must reassure her and help to instill a sense of confidence and hope while emphasizing the importance of adherence to the medicines and diet and activity instructions that he has given her. In other words, he and Renée should become partners in helping her to develop Heart Courage and to think positively.

CAD IN WOMEN

There were other aspects of Renée's case that needed attention. She is a woman with potential coronary artery or coronary heart disease who has several risk factors, including:

- A positive family history of cardiovascular disease and diabetes
- A personal history of being overweight and having uncontrolled high blood pressure
- Financial and occupational stress.

Doctors used to think that women were less susceptible to heart attacks than men, but we now know that, in fact, women are significantly more endangered by this disease than men, and their death rate is higher. Doctors often miss the diagnosis because of their misperception of lesser risk to women. So Renée's doctor must seriously consider her complaints and proceed methodically to diagnose coronary disease. In doing so, he should recognize that she might not give the classic textbook presentation of coronary disease, which was based on experiences with treating males.

In addition, Renée needs special consideration because she is an African-American woman, a group that has more risk factors and tends to have worse outcomes than other races. There is also a tendency for primary care doctors not to refer African-American women as frequently as others to cardiologists for coronary X-rays because they do not suspect them of having coronary disease.

HEART COURAGE IN MEN

What does Heart Courage in men look like? *Is* there a difference between women and men in this matter? Let us look at a typical situation. George Denunzio is a 48-year-old Caucasian bricklayer who lives in Boston with his wife and five children. He has been a blue-collar worker since he left school in the 11th grade. George likes to brag about the fact that he has never had a serious illness. Medically speaking, he comes from a good line. His parents are both in their late seventies and have never had any serious health challenges.

George enjoys life. He says his only vice is that he smokes a pack of cigarettes a day and sometimes has too many beers when he is out with the boys or watching sports on TV, which is his main pastime. George feels good about the job that he and his wife have done raising the kids. George's wife, Nancy, is a legal secretary and even though they are both working they have made a nice family environment in the home they recently purchased in a middle-class neighborhood of Medford, a Boston suburb.

George has few complaints, but he does have one. His sexual energy has dropped off tremendously, and he feels embarrassed about not being able to please his wife as much as previously. He also feels embarrassed over perceiving himself as less of a man.

Though George does not like doctors, his problem felt serious enough to cause him to make an appointment with the family physician. George hoped that his family doctor could solve his problem with pills. When the doctor asked George about his medical history, the lack of sexual energy came up. George also remembered a few other things he had been wondering about. He told the doctor that he got up several times a night to urinate and that he was much more thirsty than usual. Oh, and also he had put on more than a few extra pounds in the past two years.

After listening carefully, the doctor thanked George for this important information and began a physical examination, which included checking George's vital signs (blood pressure, heart rate, temperature, and respiratory rate), recording his height and weight, and measuring his waist. As part of the exam, the doctor did a rectal exam and checked his prostate gland.

After a complete history and physical, George's family doctor met with George and his wife in his office. "George, we have many things to discuss. We have some problems, but if we act now we can stay ahead of the game," the doctor explained. He went on to say that many of the problems he had found were treatable, and, with compliance and courage on George's part, together they could get him feeling better quickly. "So let's go slowly and discuss all the issues one at a time," the doctor said.

The doctor told George that he wanted George to see a urologist because his prostate gland was enlarged and that he may have erectile dysfunction. He went on to say that the urologists would make the definitive diagnosis and recommend treatment accordingly.

He also told George that he was extremely overweight and had high blood pressure. George's obesity was concentrated in his abdominal area, what the doctor called "visceral," or "gut," fat as opposed to the gluteus or "butt" fat pattern seen more commonly in women. The male pattern is believed to be more dangerous. It is more commonly associated with health problems such as heart disease, diabetes, and erectile dysfunction.

George also found out that his cholesterol levels and blood sugars were high. "George," the doctor explained, "you have what is called 'metabolic syndrome' and you are at a high risk of having cardiovascular disease." The doctor continued and explained to George that metabolic syndrome is the existence of several medical conditions such as high blood pressure, increased waist circumference, high sugar, and low levels of good cholesterol (HDL). "What this means George is that you are at an increased risk of having a heart attack and/or a stroke," his doctor concluded. Obviously this came as a shock to George, as he always thought a pill was all he needed to help him with his erection problem.

That seemed to be the bottom line: George was at risk of having a cardiovascular event such as a heart attack or stroke. He would have to start on medications aimed at a particular part of the syndrome. George's doctor also referred him to a cardiologist, who would look into the possibility of occult heart disease—that is, symptoms hidden to an ordinary medical examination. At this point, George had had all he could take of the doctor's tests and suspicions. He left the office still telling the doctor that he was fine, just fine, except for his erection problem. Back home it was tough for George and Nancy. They did not usually talk about health issues, especially health issues related to sex. But this time they did talk. Nancy held George and reassured him, and urged him to follow the doctor's orders. "George, this is for both of us," she told him.

But George kept worrying about his heart. He spent a lot of time now thinking about it, but in denial: "No, there can't be anything wrong with my heart!" George had always been strong and healthy. Sure, maybe he smoked too much, and maybe he drank too much beer. Okay, so he had put on a few pounds and had become a "couch potato." What has all that got to do with him developing diabetes and high blood pressure? How could he be at risk of a heart attack? Weren't his parents alive and well at ripe old ages, and had hardly ever been seriously ill? After all, the doctor could be wrong. That is what George kept saying to himself.

Nancy calmed him down and tried to reason with him. She told him that he should follow the doctor's orders, and to trust the doctor's judgment. She begged George at least to go see the cardiologist and urologist. In the meantime, she would see that he took the medicine that was prescribed and stop smoking and beer-drinking.

She also vowed to start cooking differently and they would start taking an evening walk together. They would also get more information about diabetes, high blood pressure, and heart disease.

What Nancy and George learned was how a family partnership in health worked. To begin, it involves commitment to learning more about health problems, which, untreated, could be a threat not just to the patient but also to the family. We start learning by being willing to look reality in the eye and telling ourselves the truth. Once we face the truth with courage, we are on the pathway to health and wellness.

The doctor had given George material to read about his condition. That was not enough for Nancy and George. They kept pursuing more information. There was no talk anymore of "doctor's orders." George and Nancy had become true partners with their doctor in the management of George's heart condition, if it proved he had one. George and Nancy had the courage to go to both the urologist and cardiologist. *I guess old doctor was right*

Metabolic Syndrome—(ATP III) of the National Cholesterol Education Program. As published in the Journal of the American Medical Association, 2001.

The metabolic syndrome is diagnosed when three or more of the following five risk factors are found in the same patient.

Waist circumference >40.2 inches in men or >35 inches in women

Triglyceride level $\geq$150 mg/dL

HDL cholesterol level <40 mg/dL in men or <50 mg/dL in women

Blood pressure (BP) $\geq$ 130/ $\geq$ 85 mm Hg

Blood glucose $\geq$ 100 mg/dL.

The Metabolic Syndrome diagnosis can often vary according to different sources.

after all, George told himself. George indeed had metabolic syndrome along with erectile dysfunction. The good news is that both conditions are potentially treatable if diagnosed early and patients adhere to the medical treatment plan.

George was fortunate that he found out what was wrong with him at a point where treatment was still an option. He was also fortunate in learning that the stress test, echo, and other special cardiac procedures were normal, so more extensive studies of his heart were unnecessary.

The doctor gave George prescriptions for medicines to treat each component of the metabolic syndrome that he showed symptoms of. The doctor also prescribed an automated home blood pressure monitor and explained how to use it and to keep a daily diary of the blood pressure recordings. George was also given a prescription for a safe medicine to help with his erectile dysfunction. The doctor gave him directions for finding the kind of health-exercise program George now needed to maintain.

George understood that although he was at high risk of having a heart attack or some other cardiovascular event, they had an opportunity to prevent this from occurring. The doctor assured George that they would work as partners toward their common goal of George's good health. George understood that preventive methods could keep a heart event from happening.

Men can be stoic and deny that they are ill. They see heart disease as a weakness and they may exhibit a lot of bravado in rejecting the notion that it could be affecting them. For many men heart disease feels like a loss of manliness. It is like an intruder one has not been strong enough to keep out of the house. Thinking like that leads to a machismo that can be deadly if it means waiting until it is too late for treatment to be effective.

What George, Nancy, and the doctor created was the complete opposite of machismo. Now that the doctor had earned George and Nancy's trust and had helped them to develop the courage they needed to fight heart disease, it was a cooperative action. Finally, George was past anger, resistance, and denial. He had developed Heart Courage. He was now prepared to win the biggest battle of his life.

In truth, the heart patient faces a formidable opponent—the greatest killer in the industrialized world. That is not a fight you can win by yourself. Most of us need to stand in Partnership with our doctors and loved ones in order to do what we must to get our heart health back.

So, when facing the probability or reality that you have heart disease, face it head on. Fully embrace the truth, as difficult as it may be. Have the courage to learn all that you can about the disease, and fight. Fight hard! For some, meditation and prayer are beneficial, but do not stop there. Go to the doctor and follow the medical plan provided. Have the pride and courage to learn as much as possible. Work with your doctor and choose to live.

Courage:
Calm down so that you can think clearly about what you must do to deal with the problem.

Organize a detailed plan of action with the help of your doctor. Ask your family to be members of the partnership.

Understand what is happening to you by reading, asking questions of health professionals, and viewing special programs and videos on heart attacks. This kind of information is available from organizations like the American Heart Association and the Association of Black Cardiologists (go online to www.abcardio.org, or call the Association of Black Cardiologists at 800-753-9222, and ask for their booklet, *Seven Steps to a Healthy Heart*).

Resist the temptation to just give up and "let nature take its course." You must fight back after a heart attack! It takes will and an appetite for life.

Adhere to the doctor's orders. That means complying with prescriptions and taking your medicine, and following the recommendations that he or she gives you about not smoking, exercising regularly, and avoiding excessive alcohol intake.

Go to the doctor regularly so that he or she can measure your progress. Do follow-up tests, so the doctor can adjust your medicines accordingly.

Eat wisely, based on the dietary and nutritional advice that your doctor provides. Avoid dietary binges and indiscretions.

COURAGE. It may save your life!

Chapter 2

What is Coronary Artery Disease (CAD)?

WHEN JAKE AWOKE THAT SUNDAY morning in his room, he lay in bed awhile, his hands folded under his head and grinning ear to ear. Tomorrow he would move back in with his wife and kids. Yes, he had hit bottom, and now he had won back all that he had lost. Drugs and women had cost him his family, his job and his self-respect, nearly everything except his brother Jeffrey, who never gave up on him.

As he lay in bed, Jake remembered the very worst day of his life when his wife Louisa told him, firmly, but with that note of loving care that was always part of her, "Jake, you've got to move out. I can't have you living here anymore until I can trust you again." He was being run by his bad habits and no longer trusted himself. Losing his job in his law office had been bitter, but not nearly so bitter as the loss of his wife and children. Finding himself alone for the first time in years, he rented a cheap apartment he hated from the first time he looked at it, and for a week he hardly left his room. He lay in bed back then, too, adding self-accusation to self-accusation. He was just no good, he thought, and never would be. The emotional pressure he was feeling suddenly hit him at once. At 52 years of age he just did not seem content with his life. He lived alone and was separated from his wife and kids. And though he had his daily gin martini, which usually gave him just the lift he needed, he felt uneasy and it would not go away.

Slowly Jake found out something about himself he had not known—a fire in him that refused to die. Yes, he had brought himself close to self-destruction, but he was not ready to roll into the grave through stages of worse and worse degradation. A month after Louisa threw him out, he checked himself into a recovery clinic and stayed there for several months. After outpatient work at the clinic and more than a year of therapy, Jake sent a form letter to the State Bar asking to be reinstated to practice law. The circumstances of his recovery and the confidence that his references showed in him, along with the State Bar's own meeting with Jake, convinced the Bar that Jake was a whole man again.

Today was a new day. This was the day he would meet Louisa for lunch and talk about his coming back home. Jake was feeling pretty good today, other than the slight pressure in his chest he felt from time to time. As he awaited Louisa's call, he thought about his brother Jeffrey. He needed to speak to his brother, who was a very successful surgeon, but more importantly, Jake's best friend and an excellent listener. Jake felt his life turning around and wanted to share that with his brother. Jeffrey answered the phone on the first ring. Jake shared all the good and all the bad. They had never had quite a conversation like that before. They talked for over an hour and it just felt good. Jake never told Jeffrey what he was feeling in his chest, even though Jeffrey was a doctor. Like a lot of us, Jake hated what he thought of as "whining." For him, talking about any sign of physical weakness was like whining. Instead, the brothers talked about Jake's new life, and Jake felt the warmth of his brother's love sweep over him. Jeffrey reassured Jake that everything was going to be okay now, and it was just what Jake needed to hear.

Jake knew this was true, as he lay waiting for a call from Louisa. *God has given me another shot at living my life decently,* he thought. He and Louisa would have lunch together that afternoon, and make plans for his return to her and the children on the following day. Jake had not seen much of the kids since he left home—in fact, even before that he did not see much of anything but the need to feed his bad habits. Louisa had always assured him that the kids believed he would be home soon.

The phone rang. It was Louisa. She waited on the other end, wondering why Jake was not picking up. When she got to his apartment an hour later, she found him dead.

Jake did not believe in doctors, but he had experienced warning signs, and if he had gone in for annual medical checkups, the doctor would have had the chance to recognize the signs for what they were and spelled out for Jake a treatment plan. Even before doing a physical exam, the doctor would know something about Jake's health by getting Jake's medical history, and learning that Jake's father and grandmother had died of heart disease. A family history of CAD does not mean that you too will have the disease, but in some cases it is a contributing factor. The doctor would have also discovered that Jake had several other risk factors. Jake had smoked heavily for years, a factor which, added to his heavy use of alcohol, made matters worse.

To follow what he had learned while taking Jake's medical history, the doctor would have also ordered clinical and diagnostic tests. The results, along with what he knew already, would have given the doctor a solid basis for diagnosing Jake's problem and indicating the steps they would need to take to fix it. Of course, none of this happened, because Jake "didn't like doctors."

A family history of CAD doesn't mean that you too will have the disease, but in some cases it's a contributing factor.

There are many guys like Jake who say they do not like doctors. What that often means is that they are afraid—afraid of serious illness, afraid of death. Denial came easy to Jake, because, despite his smoking and other bad habits, he had been a fine athlete for most of his life, and until the last couple years of his addictions, he had regularly worked out.

Jake's fear was so bad that, even though he had felt that pressure in his chest on and off for months, he still had not gone in for a check-up. He acted as if ignoring the symptoms would make them meaningless. Jake bet wrong, and what would have been the best day of his life became the last.

Jake's case is especially painful because he had the courage to change his life but let fear keep him from going in regularly for physical exams. He also had a brother he was close to who, if he had known of Jake's discomfort, would have made sure a heart specialist addressed Jake's symptoms. Maybe the doctor would also have told Jake that we often are not the best judges of our own health. Jake had decided there was nothing wrong with him, but he was fatally mistaken.

You are not like Jake. You are reading *The Heart of the Matter* because you want to take responsibility for your own health and have a chance to live life fully and sometimes joyfully. You know too much already to explain away symptoms ("It's just indigestion," or, "I'm too young to have CAD.") Even if the times are rough for you and you cannot afford it, you can get medical attention. Ask your local librarian to show you on the computer how to find inexpensive or free medical care. Check out your lo-

Consider the facts:

☐ Heart disease is the leading cause of death for both men and women in the United States, and is a major cause of disability.

☐ Approximately 700,000 people die of heart disease each year.

☐ According to the American Heart Association, about 550,000 new cases of heart failure are diagnosed each year.

☐ Every year, over a million people in the U.S. have a heart attack. About half of them die.

☐ Coronary Artery Disease is the number one killer of African-American men and African-American women.

☐ African-American women with coronary artery disease are more likely to die than Caucasian women who suffer from the same disease.

☐ African-American smokers with coronary disease are at higher risk of death than Caucasian-American smokers with coronary disease.

☐ The more you know about Coronary Artery Disease, the better the chances that you and your loved ones won't be killed by it.

cal health center. Persevere. We are talking about your life, and the chance to have a long and happy life should outweigh any "fear of doctors."

WHAT ALL AMERICANS
SHOULD KNOW ABOUT CAD

Statistics give us the context, but people are more interesting than numbers. So let us take a closer look at what actually happened to Jake. If Jake had seen a doctor in time, he would have learned that the pain in his chest pointed to angina. Angina is

We are talking about your life, and the chance to have a long and happy life should outweigh any "fear of doctors."

the body's way of telling us that the heart is not getting the blood it needs to function normally. It is marked by the kinds of discomfort Jake suffered—that is, a feeling of heaviness, pressure, or pain in the chest, pain that sometimes spreads to the arms or neck or jaw, or radiates to the back.

Angina results from what most of us call hardening of the arteries, and what doctors call atherosclerosis, or, more simply, coronary artery disease, or just plain coronary disease. It is not very different from a plumbing problem you might experience at home when the water flow in a pipe slows or is interrupted by calcium buildup or something that sticks at a bend in the pipe.

In the human body, what clogs the arteries is not only calcium but also fat deposits and elements like platelets. When these clogs or blockages occur in the arteries that feed the heart, symptoms of angina will occur because the supply of oxygen to the heart is restricted. Like every other organ in the body, the heart needs blood in order to function properly. If the supply of oxygen-rich blood fails, heart attacks can occur.

A heart attack occurs when small or large parts of the heart muscle die because they are not receiving nourishment. In some cases the result is death.

ANATOMY OF A HEART ATTACK

In order to understand how your heart works, you also have to understand how it is put together. This anatomy lessons begins with a simple fact: your heart is a muscle. Like all muscles it needs oxygen-enriched blood to function effectively. There are two major arteries that feed the heart blood so that it can pump:

How cholesterol forms on the wall of an artery

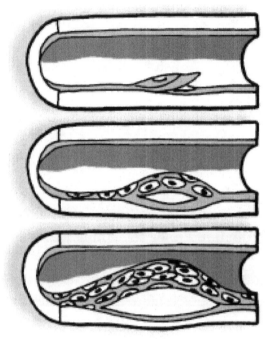

the right coronary artery and the left coronary artery. If these arteries are blocked the heart is deprived of blood. Deprived of blood, the heart, like any other muscle, suffers. That suffering can be more or less extreme. If the blood flow is decreased so that the heart starves for blood but is still sufficiently alive to function, the condition is called *ischemia,* which simply means a deficiency of blood flow. The more extreme case of heart attack, or *myocardial infarction,* means that the flow of blood has been so impaired that the heart, literally starving for blood, is dying.

Now let us look at this in a little more detail. The heart is divided into four chambers: two upper chambers and two lower ones. The upper chambers are called the *right atrium* and the *left atrium.* The lower chambers are the *right ventricle* and the *left ventricle.* Blood enters the heart through the right atrium. All the blood in the body, from the tip of your toes to the top of your head, usually passes through the right atrium.

From the right atrium, it passes to the right ventricle, the second chamber, where it is pumped into the pulmonary arteries that channel the blood up into the lungs. When we breathe, we take in oxygen that is delivered to the blood pumped from the right ventricle into our lungs. Once that blood, now enriched with oxygen, is ready to leave the lungs, it goes into the third chamber called the left atrium, and from there it goes to the left ventricle. That fourth chamber has the crucial function of pumping the blood into the *aorta*—the major blood vessel coming off the heart that supplies blood to every other artery in the body.

The aorta, because it feeds all these secondary arteries, is responsible for supplying the oxygen-rich blood and nutrients to every organ of the body. It does this by means of branches, the aorta resembling the trunk. The branches, or *arteries*, feed our muscles, tissues, and organs. This is possible through a system of *capillaries*, which are narrower tubes that transfer blood from the organs to their destinations. It is from the capillaries that the muscles, tissues, and organs extract the oxygen and nutrients they need to function properly.

Once that extraction has occurred, the blood travels from capillaries into *veins*. These veins carry the blood to the larger veins called the *superior vena cava* and the *inferior vena cava*. And, if you get the gist, you will have guessed that those large veins carry the blood back to the first chamber of the heart, the right atrium, where the process begins again.

To review, blood already drained of oxygen and nutrients comes into the heart, where it is resupplied with oxygen, then pumped through the left atrium to the left ventricle, and out through a major highway of the heart—that is, the major artery—called the aorta. The aorta disperses blood throughout the

**Decreased blood flow to heart may
cause heart muscle damage**

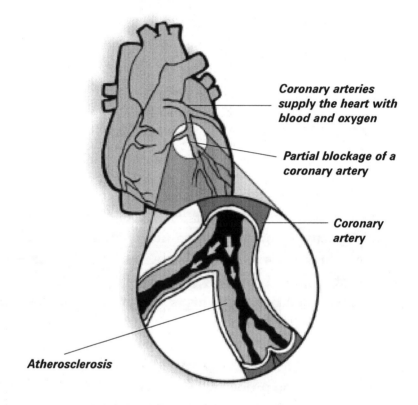

*Coronary arteries
supply the heart with
blood and oxygen*

*Partial blockage of a
coronary artery*

*Coronary
artery*

Atherosclerosis

**Coronary arteries progressively
closing (from left to right) resulting
from coronary artery disease.**

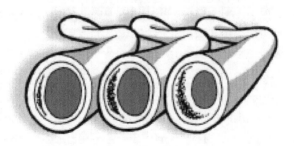

body and into smaller branches that deliver blood, by way of capillaries, to the tissues, muscles, and organs. There, the oxygenated nutrients are extracted and the blood is carried through the veins back to the right side of the heart.

There are two last details: first, coming off the aorta are two arteries—the right coronary artery and the left coronary artery. As their names indicate, the right coronary artery supplies the right side of the heart with blood and the left coronary artery supplies the left side of the heart with blood. When these arteries or their branches become clogged, the result can be angina or a heart attack.

Second, the aorta leads to two other arteries called the carotid arteries. When the carotid arteries become blocked, the result can be a stroke.

The good news is that not all, or even most, heart attacks are fatal. If you suffer one, you have a good chance of recovery if you get prompt and appropriate treatment. As with other problems, this one is far better nipped in the bud as soon *The good news is that not all, or even most, heart attacks are fatal.* as possible. Once there has been a heart attack, even if it is not fatal, damage has been done to the heart itself, and repair of and recovery from that damage is far more difficult than taking preventive measures to avoid the problem. As to the chances of recovering from a stroke, fully or partially, that depends on how much damage was done. The more serious the stroke, the more likelihood of coma or death. In the case of minor strokes, the chance for recovery is good.

HIGH BLOOD PRESSURE
AND ITS CONSEQUENCES

Of the risk factors that threaten patients (especially African Americans), hypertension is the most common and the most severe. The upside is that it is treatable. To ignore it is to buy serious trouble.

In this case, trouble comes in several forms. The first is coronary artery disease itself. As you know, that means the arteries around the heart are clogged. The second is congestive heart failure, which means that the heart is overworked and therefore weak. The third, most sadly, is stroke.

If high blood pressure is treated aggressively and not ignored, the risk of coronary artery disease, congestive heart failure, or stroke is greatly decreased. This may be the most important medical fact in this book, so let us repeat it: *Controlling your blood pressure greatly decreases your risk of suffering coronary disease, congestive heart failure and stroke.*

The higher the blood pressure, the more likely the walls of your arteries have become damaged, or inflamed. This inflammation leads to a build-up of debris—fatty deposits, cholesterol, and blood clots—that cling to the artery walls. The arteries then become narrower and can close completely or lead to dangerous blood clots, which can lead to a heart attack.

Even mild hypertension needs to be treated. Sometimes that treatment means you need to change your ways—eating differently, cutting down on salt, alcohol, and other substances that make hypertension worse. Sometimes treatment means medicine. The fact is that hypertension rarely goes away by itself.

Let us add a word here about congestive heart failure (CHF) and strokes, the two other possible consequences of hypertension. CHF means that the heart is not pumping effectively, and because it is weak, it cannot push blood out of itself in an efficient way and has to work overtime. It must pump more frequently and harder to supply blood and oxygen to the brain and the entire body. This condition leads to a heart that is overworked and enlarged.

One of the more dangerous consequences of hypertension is

How blood pressure is measured

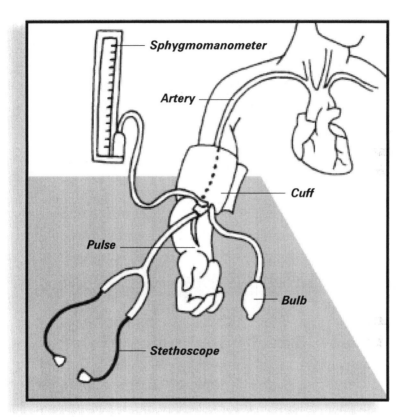

stroke. The carotid arteries carry blood to the brain. If the blood pressure in these carotid arteries is high, the artery walls become damaged and start to close, reducing the oxygen flow to the brain. This decrease of blood flow and oxygen to the brain leads to ministrokes (transient ischemic attacks or TIAs) or full-blown strokes. Because there is a decrease or stoppage of the blood flow to the brain, part of the brain itself dies.

High blood pressure is more common in African Americans than in whites and is a leading cause of early morbidity and mortality in the African-American population. Early diagnosis and treatment, along with close adherence to a medical plan, can possibly help save lives.

SYMPTOMS OF CORONARY ARTERY DISEASE

Do Not Ignore the Warning Signs

Every day hundreds of people die simply because they have ignored or did not recognize the warning signs of CAD. Do not let yourself be one of them. Though we have touched on these signs before, they bear repeating:

- Pain in the center of the chest—or, more commonly, a pressure experienced as a tightening vice or as an elephant sitting on the chest. This sensation is felt just under the breast bone, sometimes to the left side of the chest under the nipple.
- Pain in the left or right arm. Such feelings of pressure often occur while exercising, running, or working in the cold. The pain can be urgent enough to require the patient to slow down or stop what he or she is doing.
- Any chest pain or pressure that goes down the left arm or up to the throat, or jaw or back, or even to the lower back, and that lasts ten minutes or more.
- Shortness of breath
- Fast heart rate
- Nausea/vomiting
- Anxiety
- Sweating

Controlling your blood pressure greatly decreases your risk of suffering coronary disease.

While these symptoms are common to most victims of heart disease, regardless of race, studies show that African Americans are less likely to attribute the symptoms to heart problems. One may think that these symptoms could simply be the result of a bad day or plain old age—wrong! Wisdom requires that when any of these symptoms persist, they be taken seriously. Only a doctor, by an appropriate medical examination, can determine how threatening they are. The sooner the symptoms are addressed, the better the chance of early diagnosis, medical intervention, speedy recovery, and extended life.

Shortness of breath, heavy breathing, and the feeling of being hungry for air can mean that the heart is not doing its job, and can also be a sign or symptom of CAD. There are other signs that could be associated with CAD.

- Swelling of the feet or legs
- Feeling tired all the time and lacking energy
- Loss of appetite

These last signs, however, may also be associated with congestive heart failure. These symptoms of CHF mean your heart is not pumping as efficiently as it should.

The causes of CHF are various. It can simply be a late stage of coronary disease, or the result of high blood pressure or valve problems in the heart. It can also be caused by viral or bacterial infection or alcohol abuse.

Its symptoms and signs can also vary. Weight gain, shortness of breath, poor energy, and other recognized changes in the body can be indicators. Unlike coronary disease, CHF does not provide such specific symptoms as chest pain. The essential point is that coronary disease results from a blocked artery or arteries, while CHF means the heart is not working well because some of the heart muscle is dead or weak.

The most common reason for heart failure is underlying coronary disease, which is ignored by thousands who suffer from

Coronary blockage

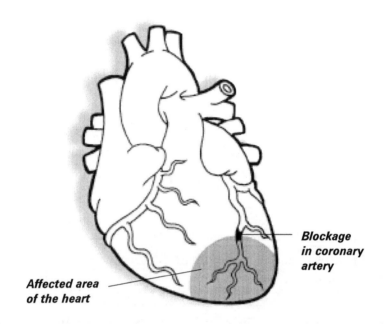

Coronary arteries feed the heart with blood. A blocked coronary, as seen above, will prevent blood from getting to this area of the heart. The heart muscle eventually dies, resulting in a heart attack or myocardial infarction (see darkened area to the right).

symptoms every day, particularly African Americans. Only a third of African Americans who suffer from the symptoms we have described will attribute them to the heart, whereas half of the white population will do so. Part of the problem is lack of knowledge—which this book was written to address. There are other problems: fear of knowing the truth; a general paranoia about doctors, nurses, hospitals, and, indeed, a deep mistrust of health care providers; and a lack of insurance or access to health facilities.

The earlier the diagnosis, the better your chances. The only way to know if the pain or discomfort you experience in the chest area is a sign of coronary disease is to get a complete medical workup—that is, a complete medical examination, including an EKG, a chest x-ray, the appropriate blood work or other lab work, and/or invasive or noninvasive cardiac testing. Such a procedure often means the difference between life and death. Lack of knowledge, poor access to health facilities, and paranoia among African Americans—though they can have real social and economic causes—have too often led to inadequate treatment, treatment that comes too late, and deaths that could have been avoided. Let us change that—starting here, starting now.

MYOCARDIAL ISCHEMIA

We have discussed this previously, but let us review again before closing. The condition in which the heart does not receive enough blood is called *myocardial ischemia*.

The earlier the diagnosis, the better your chances.

The medical term means simply that the heart muscle is not getting enough blood. Untreated myocardial ischemia can lead to heart attacks (myocardial infarction), sudden death, and congestive heart failure.

In some cases (10 to 20 percent), ischemia is "silent"—that is, the patient experiences none of the usual symptoms such as angina. Angina can be stable or unstable. When it is stable, it is predictable. For example, exertion will always bring pain, and resting will always stop it. Unstable angina is more dangerous. It is also more likely to lead to a heart attack.

These distinctions are not essential to the patient. What is important is that he or she recognize the symptoms and seek appropriate care.

Heart attacks can present as sudden death. The heart goes into a dangerous arrhythmia (irregular beat) and then stops. It is this kind of heart attack that is most publicized by the media, and that is unfortunate. The wide publicity given to such cases, with all their drama, has encouraged a kind of fatalism. People read or watch accounts of such cases and go away thinking, "See, nothing can be done. If it's going to happen, it's going to happen." That is one way we rationalize not taking care of ourselves.

The truth is that heart attacks usually follow warnings in the form of angina symptoms. Angina, when diagnosed and treated appropriately, usually has a good prognosis.

Now you know the hard facts that could have saved Jake's life if he also had known them. Now you have taken a big step away from sharing Jake's fate. We, the doctors who have written this book, have heard all the excuses. Besides simply being afraid of the truth, people think, as Jake did: "It can't happen to me. I'm an athlete in good condition." Or, "Well, if it happens, it's fate, or God's will. There's nothing I can do about it." Or, "Look at how doctors and hospitals have treated African Americans, Hispanics, and women in the past. I don't trust them." And a hundred others: "It's only indigestion," or "I'm too young." "My family, which worries about my health, is over-reacting." Or simply, "Well, I'll have it looked into later. Right now, most of the time I feel just fine."

> *The truth is that heart attacks usually follow warnings in the form of angina symptoms. And angina, when diagnosed and treated appropriately, usually has a good prognosis.*

Do not kid yourself into the grave. Have an ounce of courage and a pound of pride and, knowing what you know, see a doctor at once if you are experiencing any of the symptoms we have described.

Go to the doctor!

Chapter 3

Early Detection of Coronary Artery Disease

BY NOW YOU HAVE READ that coronary artery disease, or CAD, is the greatest killer of Americans. Each year, more than a third of the deaths that occur in the United States are caused by CAD, which, though it primarily affects people in middle to old age, also occurs frequently at younger ages. A heart attack occurs every 26 seconds in this country, and someone dies from one every minute. Fifty percent of men and 64 percent of women had no symptoms before their heart attack suddenly killed them. Though CAD occurs in both genders, each year more women than men die of heart attacks. Though CAD affects all races and ethnicities, it is disproportionately lethal in African Americans.

Medical science has made great inroads into the impact of CAD on the American population in the past three decades, but despite advances that increase a doctor's ability to prevent, diagnose, and treat CAD, it still remains more deadly than stroke, cancer, HIV/AIDS, violence, and in fact, all other causes of death.

Catching risk factors early helps some people avoid disease and others to get the most effective treatment, which is *early*

Doctors have come to recognize that the patient is the center of the medical universe, and that all of the elements in that universe revolve around him or her.

treatment. You know by now that such risk factors include hypertension, diabetes, cigarette smoking, obesity, and high blood cholesterol.

We also know that there are genetic factors that predispose certain individuals to the development of CAD. Although this progress in medical detection and research has had great benefits in the way of early detection leading to better health and longer life, there is another even more important method for the detection of CAD—you! Doctors have come to recognize that the patient is the center of the medical universe, and that all of the elements in that universe revolve around him or her. This is especially true regarding the detection of CAD. The information you give your doctor about symptoms you are experiencing, or signs that the doctor sees during your annual checkup are important tools he has to work with. Let us examine why.

Evidence suggests that CAD can be present at an early age. Autopsies performed on soldiers killed in the Korean War showed that many of these young men, some in their teens, already had signs of arteriosclerosis, or, more precisely, atherosclerosis, or fatty streaks, in their arteries. These fatty streaks are considered the first stage of CAD.

This observation, discovered by Dr. Renu Virmani and her research team at the Armed Forces Institute of Pathology in Bethesda, Maryland, several years ago, uncovered the earliest known "starting point" for the damaging process of atherosclerosis within our systems. As we first learned through this research, atherosclerosis can be compared to a time bomb inside our bodies that builds up strength until it explodes.

But in looking around at all of the seemingly healthy adults in the country, how can we tell who carries this time bomb? People who are suffering from the early stages of CAD do not usually develop any outward symptoms of the disease process going on inside them. CAD does not publicize its early presence.

CAD is not the only illness that starts early but reveals itself slowly, or even hides altogether. High blood pressure, high blood cholesterol, diabetes, and kidney disease all work in more or less the same way, silently developing before they make trouble. The doctor is left acting like a medical detective whose assignment is to make a preemptive strike on CAD before it hits you with a cardiovascular event that could be fatal.

In the early stages of CAD, doctors sometimes have no specific symptoms with which to work. Instead, they rely on what research has told them are indicators—that is, indicators that suggest you are moving toward a more threatening stage of CAD. One of these indicators is body weight, or more precisely, body mass index (BMI), which is a ratio of weight to height.

A BMI can show that you are overweight or obese and should be taken seriously. A high BMI is a risk factor for CAD just like diabetes, hypertension, and high blood cholesterol. To make matters worse, overweight children often become obese adults. Since 1970, overweight in children ages two to five has doubled; in children ages six to nineteen, it has tripled. By 2035, an estimated 100,000 cases of CAD could result from the increase in overweight and obesity—cases that need not have occurred if people paid attention to their BMI and other risk factors.

For the adult American population in general (there are some variations among genders and ethnic groups), we calculate a BMI less than 18.45 as underweight, from 18.5 to 24.9 as normal, from 25 to 29.9 as overweight, and anything over 30 as obesity.

You can calculate your own BMI online by using the calculator provided by the Centers for Disease Control and Prevention (CDC) of the U.S. Department of Health and Human Services. http://www.cdc.gov/widgets/BMIForAdults. If you do not have a computer, your local librarian can help you. The calculation does not even take a minute. You just plug your height and weight into the online calculator. There is a separate calculator for children. http://apps.nccd.cdc.gov/dnpabmi.

How reliable an indicator is BMI? *The New England Journal of Medicine* reported a study made in Denmark in which subjects had been followed from childhood for 46 years. Calculation of their BMI in childhood revealed a positive association of high BMI with coronary disease that was strongest in boys ages seven to thirteen and in girls

Since 1970, overweight in children ages two to five has doubled. In children ages six to nineteen, it has tripled.

ten to thirteen, and this association increased with age. It was stronger for boys than for girls. What this may mean is that an elevated BMI in childhood could be an indicator of future CAD. Put another way, if your children are overweight in childhood, they could be at increased risk of developing CAD as an adult. Knowing this, you must do everything possible to eliminate this threat in your children as well as in yourself. Forewarned is forearmed.

EARLY WARNINGS

Okay, you know you are overweight, but you have been enjoying good health and do not want to make changes in your eating or activity habits. When you were young you were athletic, though in the past twenty years you have made a policy of avoiding unnecessary motions. Why walk when you can drive?

Why climb stairs when there is an elevator?

Then your closest friend experiences a heart attack, and it is nearly a year before she fully recovers. You have trusted your body to take care of itself, but now you wonder: that weight you have been carrying so cheerfully—might it be a threat to your health, even to your life? So you start looking into the matter. Are there early signs to look for that might serve as early warning signals— something like that light on your dashboard that tells you your car needs a checkup?

In fact there are. The first indication of CAD for many is **chest pain,** which doctors have been calling by its Latin name, *angina pectoris,* for roughly 300 years. You have learned when your heart is not getting enough blood (myocardial ischemia) the heart cries out in pain. This pain is called angina. Angina is usually located in the front and center of the chest, just beneath the breastbone or to the left or right of center. However, it may also be felt in other areas of the body, such as in the jaw, arm, or back. It may radiate or travel down the left arm, up the neck, or into the back.

If your children are overweight in childhood, they could be at increased risk of developing CAD as an adult.

Angina usually occurs with increased activity. The pain may come when you are active but it can also occur when you are at rest. It may even awaken you from sleep, which is a particularly ominous sign.

Angina is often described as a crushing pain, like someone has reached inside of your chest and is squeezing your heart. Patients may demonstrate this by holding their balled-up fist in front of their chest. Some people say that severe angina feels "like an elephant is sitting on my chest."

Angina can also be mistaken as indigestion or "gas pains." Often, people try to relieve this distress with antacids, usually with poor results. Others describe a sensation that is like a knife stab. Some people do not experience CAD as pain so much as a "misery"—that is, an uncomfortable feeling hard to describe.

To confuse the picture even more, not everyone experiences the complaints just described. CAD can announce itself with the sudden occurrence of shortness of breath, profuse sweating, dizziness or being light-headed, nausea, vomiting, and palpitations, these last described as a racing of the heart and a sensation of the heart doing "flip-flops" inside the chest. The sensation may be caused by a disturbance of the regular heart beat (arrhythmias)—another serious warning sign.

Let us look at a scenario to illustrate what can happen when a person develops CAD. Frank Bidler is a 45-year-old Caucasian dentist. He lives with his wife, Loretta, and two children in an upscale suburb of Phoenix, Arizona. He prides himself on taking good care of himself and his family.

Frank has always been in good health (except for what he calls "a little bit of high blood pressure"). His family doctor has told him to always take his high blood pressure medications. Frank knows what that means and does what he can to comply. He plays golf twice a week with a group of buddies, avoids things known to damage his health (he does not smoke, and drinks only a glass or two of his beloved single-malt scotch on the rocks about three times a week), gets proper rest (he sleeps an average of five or six hours a night— adequate, he feels, under the circumstances of family and professional demands), avoids stress (he and his wife go to the movies a couple of times a month, and they and the kids take an annual week-long vacation), and eats healthy foods (he avoids fast food and eats a couple of vegetables with dinner, although he cannot resist the prime steaks or succulent chops that they enjoy about twice a week, and he uses a tad of salt on those delectable home fries, but tries to be careful with it).

Lately, however, Frank has found that the movies and a weeklong vacation are not enough to keep his stress under control. He feels money pressures and works longer and longer hours, and lately he has had less energy when he comes home from the office. He has also been drinking a little more regularly in the evening. "Scotch helps me to de-stress," he says, and he jokes that it "keeps me from distress." Frank is an optimistic and focused man. He is not too concerned about how he has been feeling lately. *This too shall pass,* he thought.

Then one morning as Frank got out of bed he felt what he calls a "twinge" of pain right beneath his breastbone, and, at the same time, a very rapid beating of his heart. He got back in bed and after two or three minutes the pain went away. But when he got up ten minutes later the pain came back, along with the rapid heartbeat.

Frank did not worry too much about these discomforts. *I probably ate too much of that delicious spaghetti and meatballs that Loretta fixed last night,* he thought. He took an Alka-Seltzer Plus® before breakfast and was convinced that this would do the trick.

Some people do not experience CAD as pain so much as a "misery"—that is, an uncomfortable feeling hard to describe.

The next night while he was watching Monday Night Football the same symptoms returned, but this time the pain was stronger—*five on a scale of one-to-ten,* he thought, and it lasted longer. Frank, though he was sitting still, found himself sweating. That is when he started worrying and finally told Loretta about what he was feeling.

Loretta immediately swung into action. Over Frank's faint protests, she called 911 and told them she thought her husband was having a heart attack and to send help. Then she crushed two aspirin tablets for him to swallow. The paramedics arrived within ten minutes and checked Frank's blood pressure, which was elevated, and his heart rate, which was fast and irregular. They did an electrocardiogram (EKG) that revealed evidence of myocardia ischemia and rapid heart beats.

The paramedics started an intravenous drip and called in to the base doctor at the hospital emergency room, who reviewed the EKG that they transmitted electronically. He instructed them to give him a "clot-buster" drug and to transport Frank with a heart monitor attached.

When Frank arrived in the ER, the doctor saw him immediately and repeated the EKG. Compared to the first one, it showed that the heart had settled down, but the diagnosis was acute coronary syndrome (ACS)—that is, a true cardiac emergency. The EM doctor drew some blood for determination of cardiac enzymes that are released when heart cells are damaged, and also ordered several other tests to be done in the laboratory,

---

Perhaps nothing we say in this book is of greater potential importance to you than the following:

☐ If you think you are suffering a heart attack, take two aspirins, crushed, and call 911. Stay calm.

☐ Do not call your doctor or the local hospital—just call 911.

☐ Do not even attempt to drive yourself and do not let your loved ones drive. Wait for the ambulance to come. That way you will get treated faster during the early stages of the heart attack and have a better chance at survival.

☐ If the attack is happening to someone else, call 911. There is no time for denial or for lengthy discussion. Life is hanging on a thread.

highest priority.

The doctor continued the drip of the clot buster drug and had Frank admitted to the Coronary Care Unit (CCU) of the hospital. There they continued to do diagnostic studies and treatment. When the test reports came back the doctor told Frank that he had not had a classic heart attack, or myocardial infarction. What Frank experienced was acute coronary insufficiency. That meant that there had been a build up of "plaque," made up of cholesterol and other substances, inside one of the arteries that supply blood and oxygen to his heart muscle, blocking the blood and oxygen supply. Specifically, the plaque in Frank's coronary artery ruptured, leading to clot formation and this clot blocked blood flow in the artery itself. Rapid administration of aspirin and the clot-busting drug had helped to reopen the artery.

Frank was also given a coronary angiogram, a procedure that involves inserting a long tube or catheter into the heart through a leg artery. The coronary arteries are then injected with dye, allowing the doctors to see the blockage and to clear the blockage by inserting a small balloon inside the coronary artery (angioplasty). This procedure also involved permanent placement in the artery of a small rigid tube called a stent, which keeps the artery open. These procedures, along with some very important medicines, could help Frank avoid having a heart attack in the future.

THE IMPORTANCE OF
EARLY DETECTION OF CAD

What message does Frank's case deliver about the importance of early detection of CAD? It should tell you that a heart attack can occur in anyone, even in a person who appears healthy. Knowing this, you must prepare yourself, as Loretta had, to recognize the early warning signs of heart problems. Angina, as in Frank's case, sends a clear signal that something is not quite right inside your chest and that you need to take steps immediately to protect your heart or a loved one's. The more you delay when that first warning occurs, the greater the potential damage to your heart. As cardiologists put it, "time is muscle," meaning that immediate action must be taken when that twinge of pain that you thought was indigestion occurs. Of course, you may be wrong, it may not be a heart attack, but it is better to be wrong than to be sorry.

Frank was lucky that his delay did not result in disablement or even death. He was also lucky that his wife Loretta had learned how to deal with an acute cardiac event when she attended a weekend health fair. That is where she learned about the warning signs and about using the aspirin and calling 911 right away. Now, she and Frank and the kids have all taken a course in cardiopulmonary resuscitation or CPR, and the whole family has undergone a *total lifestyle change* in which they eat heart-healthy foods, are mindful of their BMI and understand that a high BMI can be a risk factor for CAD events. They also exercise regularly, even Frank, who understands that exercise has to be one of his highest priorities and that he must make time for it. Finally, they all have learned ways of managing stress and avoiding unnecessary stress. They take time to relax and get adequate rest and sleep.

Though still in the experimental phase, there are some new technological tools in the works that may help alert the patient to the fact that he or she is having a heart attack. One is a Bluetooth-like monitor the patient wears that works through a cell phone, which actually calls the patient when an abnormal EKG or arrhythmia is detected. Another device uses a global positioning system or GPS similar to the one in some cars, which is linked to a satellite orbiting the earth. It has the potential of not only monitoring the patient but also pinpointing his or her location and alerting both patient and hospital. These types of devices are expected to be more valuable for use in patients who have already had a heart attack, not someone like Frank in our scenario above. We are not completely there yet with these "space-age" novelties. For now, you have to rely on yourself and your team of healthcare providers to be the sentinel of your own survival.

Remember that although you should always work with your doctor when you have a heart challenge, your life is basically in YOUR hands!!

Cardiologists talk about the "golden hour," the time from the moment heart attack symptoms begin to the moment when serious, perhaps irreversible damage and even death may occur. This is the optimal time for doctors to do their best to save your life. Obviously, the faster you spring into action when you get that first symptom, the better your chances of survival will be.

Remember that although you should always work with your doctor when you have a heart challenge, your life is basically in YOUR hands!! You now know that a healthy diet, exercise, and reducing stress can keep you on the path of maintaining a healthy heart. Do not let your life slip through your fingers!!

Chapter 4

Heart Disease
in Women
New Evidence, New Thinking,
Brighter Future

MARY AND HER HUSBAND, both middle-aged, had been see-ing their doctor for the past five years. They were both usually upbeat and determined people, but today's visit was different. Mary appeared frightened and distracted. For a while she did what she could to cover her mood, but finally, she said, "Doctor, I've always thought that breast cancer was a woman's greatest health risk, but just this past year one of my close friends suffered a sudden heart attack, another need-ed bypass surgery, and one died suddenly when her heart just stopped. I feel like I'm walking in a mine field." Mary talked about all this with her head down, her eyes on the floor. She continued, "I always thought that heart disease was a threat to men but not to women. Now I'm beginning to wonder."

Her doctor replied with the hard facts, which startled Mary:

- Coronary heart disease (CHD also known as CAD) is the leading cause of death for women in the United States.
- One in nine women aged 45–64 years has coronary

disease; this rate increases to one in three for women older than 65.

- While it is true that women develop CHD ten years later than men, in general, the prognosis for women is worse. Women suffer more complications, they are more likely to die, and both bypass surgery and angioplasty are less successful in women.

Even after she heard these facts, Mary had a hard time letting go of her convictions: "But I thought this was a 'man's' disease that I didn't have to worry about."

"No, Mary," the doctor explained. "Maybe the reason people get that false impression is that women in general report symptoms of heart disease to a doctor about ten years later than men. The fact remains that after menopause the rapid increase in CAD and death rates for women make them about the same as those for a man. In fact, since 1984, each year more women than men have died from heart disease."

We know from experience and from reading studies that Mary's misconceptions are widely shared. A Gallup poll conducted in 1995 by the American Medical Women's Association and the American Heart Association found that 80% of the women surveyed did not know that heart disease is the leading cause of death in American women. Even more surprising, 32% of doctors in the same poll did not know it either. The idea that women do not get heart disease is deeply ingrained in our society.

Mary had been through a stunning experience during her ten minutes in the doctor's office. Strong woman that she was, her mind had been changed, so she kept asking questions: "I've just recently gone through menopause," she said. "I read somewhere that hormone replacement therapy reduces a woman's risk of heart disease. Is that true? Should I be taking that?" This was a good question to ask. The doctor went on to provide Mary with more facts.

Hormone replacement therapy (HRT) for the prevention of CHD in women was a routine recommendation until 1994, when a new study changed that. The Heart and Estrogen/Progestin Replacement Study (HERS) trial conducted in women with known heart disease showed strong evidence that treatment with combined HRT (estrogen + progesterone) did *not* reduce deaths from heart disease. In fact, this particular hormone replacement therapy may have been associated with an early increased risk of death. Mary was shocked to learn this.

In women without a history of heart disease, the Women's Health Initiative Study showed that combined HRT was worse than just being ineffective in decreasing deaths from CHD. The treatment was also associated with an increased risk of cardiovascular events—that is, of heart problems of every kind.

The HRT trial was stopped early due to clear harm to the group of patients participating in the clinical trial. The Women's Health Initiative Estrogen Alone study showed that estrogen used alone also did not protect against CHD, although this study showed no evidence that it did harm. This data completely changed the recommendations for hormone replacement therapy in postmenopausal women to prevent heart disease.

Currently, the major medical organizations state that there is *no* role for hormone replacement therapy in the prevention of heart disease, and that hormone replacement therapy should be used only for the relief of menopausal symptoms (such as hot flashes), and even then only for the shortest time necessary to control these symptoms.

The doctor's answer to Mary's question was simply, no, there was no miracle treatment to give her. Mary would have to take charge of her own health, with her doctor's guidance.

The doctor went on to explain that conditions or predispositions that may lead to a disease are called "risk factors." She reminded Mary that she had several risk factors. "Your mother died of heart disease, and we've had to monitor your cholesterol and blood pressure lately. I'd say we've come to the point where you have to make some lifestyle changes."

"What changes would those be?" Mary asked.

"Healthy eating is important," her doctor explained. "A healthy diet includes plenty of fruits and vegetables, lowering or cutting out salt, and eating less saturated fat and cholesterol. I'll give you pamphlets later with more detail about diet and about why salt and saturated fats are dangerous."

"Another thing you should be doing, which we're already taking care of, is monitoring your blood pressure and cholesterol levels. Those are both risk factors, and from last week's tests I see the situation isn't improving. A lot of people at your stage are walking around with heart problems they don't know they have because they never go visit a doctor."

All adults over 40 who do not have risk factors should have their blood pressure and cholesterol checked at least once every five years. Those who do or might have risk factors, and the elderly, should be monitored more often. Obviously, this means not waiting until you are sick to go in for a medical examination. Even if you are young and in the best of health, the examination and tests will be reference points for down the line. Remember, with heart disease, as with many other conditions, the earlier it gets spotted the more effective treatment is likely to be.

"So you're doing an important thing, Mary. You're coming in to see me even when you aren't ill—that is, you schedule regular health checkups."

Mary's doctor also recommended that Mary make another change besides eating a healthier diet—more exercise. Walking more, even up and down stairs, maybe just a flight or two to start, will jumpstart Mary's exercise routine.

Every able person should engage in at least moderate physical activity for at least thirty minutes on most days of the week to maintain a healthy weight. Even if you are not in full good health, your doctor or physical therapist will usually recommend some exercise that you can do and feel better for doing. Remember that the heart is a muscle and, like any muscle, it needs exercise to work strongly and efficiently. Working out at least three times a week at a local gym or Y is also helpful.

Remember that the heart is a muscle and, like any muscle, it needs exercise to work strongly and efficiently.

Sure, it can be hard to start, but once you get into the routine, you may find it difficult to stop.

A combination of healthy diet with regular exercise is the best prescription of all. Eating healthier helps us to restrict the calories in our diet. Exercise helps us to burn calories. It is widely recognized that physical activity reduces the risk for heart disease and that walking is an excellent form of exercise. In one analysis of data from the Nurses' Health Study, researchers obtained detailed information on physical activity from 72,488 women, aged 40 to 65. During eight years of follow-up, 645 women developed heart disease.

The study established that there is a significant relationship between the amount of physical activity we do and our risk of developing heart disease. Those with the highest activity level had 44% lower risk of developing heart disease than those with the lowest amount of physical activity. Interestingly, the benefit of walking was similar to that gained from more vigorous types of exercise. As little as an hour a week has benefits. Once you get into the habit of walking, if you are like most, you will enjoy it and will want to do more.

"So that's your menu, Mary," her doctor said. "The payoff isn't just that you'll be healthier and live longer, but also that nearly everyone who tries it says that the combination of exercise and good eating habits makes them feel good, physically and emotionally. That's just as certain as people who smoke or abuse drug are at greater risk of CAD."

Mary managed to get through most of the discussion attentively. It was a lot to take in. She was worried about her heart and she took the recommendations in and was ready for more. Although women with heart disease have pretty much the same risk factor profiles as men, the connection between having a risk factor and getting the disease may differ between men and women. Let us look at smoking for example.

In the past several decades, the percentage of people smoking cigarettes has declined. The decline, however, has been much more dramatic in men (21% decrease) than in women (6% decrease). Furthermore, while smoking among women overall has declined, the incidence of cigarette smoking among *young* women has actually increased. Twenty-five percent of women still smoke, although smoking is one of the major risk factors for heart disease occurring in pre-menopausal women.

Younger women seem to be particularly vulnerable to the effects of cigarette smoking, and the risk appears to depend on the dose. The danger of heart disease is related to the number of cigarettes a woman smokes a day, although smoking as few as one to four cigarettes per day raises the risk of dying from heart disease more than two-fold.

If you do smoke, STOP. Despite advertising to the contrary, low-nicotine and filtered cigarettes do not decrease the risk associated with smoking. The good news, according to current research, is that stopping smoking can reduce the risk of heart disease by more than 50% within two years. So the message is clear: if you do not smoke, do not start. If you do smoke, STOP.

Smoking was not Mary's concern. Mary had recently developed high cholesterol, and though she was taking a medication for that, medicines best help those who help themselves. Before age 20, men and women have similar cholesterol levels; from 20 to 55, men tend to have higher total cholesterol levels than women, but after 55 years of age, women's cholesterol levels increase rapidly and may slightly exceed those of men.

Women's levels of high-density lipoprotein cholesterol (HDL—the "good" cholesterol) are typically higher than those of men, and they remain higher throughout much of life. But absolute levels of HDL decline following menopause, and from that point on HDL levels are about the same between the sexes. Pre-menopausal women have lower triglyceride levels than men and postmenopausal women; however, with aging, triglyceride levels increase more in women than they do in men. (Triglycerides are a type of fat that occur in the blood and that, at high enough levels, can clog arteries.)

As is true for men, increased LDL ("bad") cholesterol, decreased HDL ("good") cholesterol, and increased triglyceride levels are risk factors for heart disease in women. HDL and triglyceride levels, in fact, appear to be even more powerful risk factors for women than for men.

In women with high heart disease risk, cholesterol-lowering medications (such as statins) help reduce heart attacks, strokes and total mortality. (See appendix for more information on statins). This was demonstrated in several research studies, including one called the Cholesterol and Recurrent Events (CARE) study. The CARE study evaluated 4,159 subjects with prior myocardial infarction (heart attack) but only modestly elevated cholesterol levels, and found that after five years of treatment with a statin, both men and women had fewer cardiovascular events. We know that these statistics can get a bit heavy, but the more you know, the better you can protect yourself from heart disease.

By this point of her visit, Mary had learned much more than she had expected. She never thought her doctor would take the time to explain how to maintain a healthy heart, particularly because she herself was not ill and had just come in for a checkup. Mary was smart. She took this time to get as much information as possible. In addition to her cholesterol levels, the things that concerned Mary most were high blood pressure, diabetes, and her weight. Her doctor explained that all played a part in developing heart disease.

"Unfortunately, not enough women and men are getting hypertension treatment," her doctor said. "Control of hypertension reduces the risk of stroke or death in both men and women, and in those with only mild hypertension as well as those with severe hypertension.

"Hypertension is less common in younger women, but it appears to be even more dangerous when it does occur. Premenopausal women with hypertension are ten times more likely to die of coronary heart disease than young women without hypertension."

The information Mary received was tough to swallow, but she did not let her fear deter her. After all, she had come this far.

The doctor continued and told Mary that diabetes is an even more powerful risk factor for heart disease in women than it is for men. One study found that men with diabetes were nearly two-and-a-half times more likely to develop heart disease over men without diabetes. The Nurses' Health Study reported a 6.3-fold increased risk for cardiovascular mortality among women with diabetes than among those without.

This study also found that even if a woman had been diagnosed with diabetes for fewer than four years, the risk of heart disease was significantly elevated. The reasons for this markedly increased risk among women with diabetes are not completely understood. However, it may be at least in part due to the fact that diabetes is usually associated with other cardiac risk factors such as obesity, hypertension, low HDL and high triglycerides.

We all have friends who walk around with these conditions without realizing their seriousness. As Mary learned, several risk factors for heart disease can be prevented or even corrected by changes in diet and physical activity. The same is true of diabetes.

Diabetes is an even more powerful risk factor for heart disease in women than it is in men.

So remember, when it comes to your health, practice prevention. It is your body, your life. Do not leave it entirely in the hands of doctors to fix what is ailing you or to keep you from getting ill. Some of the factors that will determine how long and how healthy a life you will lead are in *your* hands.

Unfortunately, some are not. In one study of young women with heart disease, the most common cardiac risk factor was a family history of premature heart disease (67%), followed by smoking (55%) and high cholesterol (55%). Nonetheless, changing your habits is a small price to pay for living longer, and for just plain feeling strong and good.

Mary had been taking notes all through the run-down of risks and preventive measures. The real issue had not been addressed. She had gained nearly twenty pounds since she left high school and she was worried about her weight. Although she had tried several diet plans, none of them worked for her in the long run. The risk of heart disease increases as people

*Do not leave it en-
tirely in the hands of
doctors to fix what is
ailing you or to keep
you from getting ill.*

become more overweight. A weight gain of ten pounds or more after the age of eighteen is considered a risk factor.

A few recent studies have given us a little insight into the short-term benefits of some popular diets, though not the longterm benefits. One recent study compared the Atkins, Zone, Ornish and Weight Watchers diets for weight loss and for cardiac risk factors in 160 patients, 40 patients per group, with an average weight of 220 pounds at the start of the study.

All of the diets resulted in modest weight loss over 12 months, with no significant difference between diets. Most strikingly, all diets had a positive effect on cardiac risk factors, with an increase in HDL and decrease in LDL cholesterol and insulin levels. Interestingly, the diets with the more severe restrictive patterns— Atkins and Ornish— had the highest dropout rates. What is clear is that even modest weight loss has a positive impact on cardiovascular health. And you will obviously help that slimming-down process if you add regular exercise to your diet routine.

After her discussion with the doctor, Mary was visibly relieved, and she now understood that much of heart disease is preventable and that she can do so many things to lower her heart disease risk. She plans to start today, with changes for herself, her husband and her entire family. **What changes will you make today?**

Chapter 5

Lifestyle Choices
to Prevent
Heart Disease

FRANK WEDGEWORTH, a 51-year-old African-American male, visited his doctor as a new patient for a general health checkup. Frank believed he was fairly healthy, but his father had died suddenly of a heart attack at the age of 55 and Frank worried that his own health had suffered over the past few years from lack of exercise and increased work stress. He works as a manager of a department store—the same store that he had been working at for over 20 years, beginning as a salesman and rising over the years to a managerial position with a desk job.

Frank had been physically active in his youth. He played most sports and had even played college basketball for a short time. His wife, too, had been athletic, and when they first got married, they loved to take walks together and to play sports. As they began having children and their jobs got more demanding, their physical activity diminished. Frank did not know how much weight he had gained over the years, but he knew that his belt size had increased and he has had to buy his clothes in a larger size.

Frank was prompted to see a cardiologist because he was

recently diagnosed with borderline high blood pressure ("pre-hypertension" his physician called it), and he was now close to the age at which his father died. Frank realized that it was time to take better control of his health. "Our bodies have always taken care of us," he said to Alicia, his wife; "now maybe it's time for us to take care of our bodies."

Hypertension (high blood pressure) strikes people of color more often, at younger ages, and with more severe complications than it strikes other populations.

Upon his visit, Frank was congratulated on being ready to make healthy lifestyle changes. He was reminded that cardiovascular diseases (diseases of the heart and blood vessels) kill almost a million Americans each year, and that up to 80% of these deaths are preventable by simple lifestyle changes. Today, doctors talk a lot about what puts people at risk for heart disease—they call these warning signs "cardiovascular risk factors." Some of these factors are:

- A family history of early heart disease
- High blood pressure
- High blood cholesterol level, particularly a high LDL-cholesterol level (LDL is sometimes known as the "bad" cholesterol)
- Low HDL-cholesterol level (HDL is sometimes referred to as the "good" cholesterol)
- Cigarette smoking
- Diabetes mellitus
- Lack of physical activity
- Obesity
- Increasing age
- Being male, or being a post-menopausal female

Frank asked for specific information on how he could help to lower his blood pressure with lifestyle changes. According to the National Institute of Health, a normal blood pressure is less than 120/80 mm Hg. The top number (the 120) is called the "systolic blood pressure;" the bottom number (the 80) is called the "diastolic blood pressure." Frank's blood pressure was 135/85. He was considered pre-hypertensive.

Hypertension (high blood pressure) strikes people of color more often, at younger ages, and with more severe complications than it strikes other populations. Because high blood pressure threatens the health of the heart, it needs to be treated. While medications help, treatment of hypertension should begin with lifestyle changes. These include weight reduction for those who are overweight, moderation of alcohol intake, increased physical activity, reduction in sodium (salt) intake, adequate intake of dietary potassium, adequate intake of dietary calcium, and cessation of smoking.

Since Frank wanted to know what diet changes he needed to make, he was told about the DASH (Dietary Approaches to Stop Hypertension) and DASH-Sodium trials, which conclusively demonstrated that managing one's diet can reduce blood pressure. These studies demonstrated that a diet low in saturated fat, cholesterol, salt, and total fat, and high in fruits, vegetables, and low-fat dairy foods reduce blood pressure.

The DASH trial studied 459 patients, 60% of whom were African Americans. Patients were assigned to one of three diets:

- The "control" diet, which had levels of fat and cholesterol that matched the average American's diet.
- The "fruit and vegetable" diet, which matches the control diet in fat, saturated fat, cholesterol, and protein. The only difference between them is that potas-

sium, magnesium, and fiber got a boost when fruits and vegetables replaced some snacks and sweets.

- The "combination" diet, which had less total fat, saturated fat, and cholesterol than the fruit and vegetable diet or the control diet, and was also rich in fruits, vegetables, and low-fat dairy products (which increased the potassium, magnesium, calcium, fiber, and protein content of the diet).

The results: systolic blood pressure (the top number) decreased by 5.5 mm Hg and diastolic blood pressure (the bottom number) decreased 3.0 mm Hg in people on the combination diet as compared with people on the control diet. The effect was even greater among African Americans (6.9/3.7 mm Hg reductions). Furthermore, among those with the highest blood pressures to begin with, the reductions in systolic and diastolic blood pressure were 11.4 and 5.5 mm Hg, and these blood pressure reductions were evident within two weeks.

The DASH-Sodium study was designed to evaluate the effect of different levels of dietary sodium (salt), in conjunction with the DASH diet, on blood pressure. This study included 412 patients (57% African American). Patients were randomly assigned to a DASH or a control diet for one month at each of three salt levels (1,500, 2,400, or 3,300 mg/day). The reductions in blood pressure were greatest among those on the DASH diet with the lowest so-

Although drugs like statin medications for high cholesterol and procedures like angioplasty are critical in the overall treatment of heart disease, diet and lifestyle therapies remain the foundation of efforts to prevent cardiovascular disease.

dium intake of 1,500 mg/day. Systolic blood pressure was further reduced by 11.5 mm Hg in patients on the DASH diet and a low level of sodium, as against those on the control diet and a high level of sodium. The effect was even greater among African-American patients (12.6 mm Hg difference).

Although drugs like statin medications for high cholesterol and procedures like angioplasty are critical in the overall treatment of heart disease, diet and lifestyle therapies remain the foundation of efforts to prevent cardiovascular disease. As Frank began to recognize steps he could take to help himself, he became more and more eager to begin. He asked for a point-by-point rundown of preventive strategies. His doctor was happy to share the following information with him.

Instituting healthy dietary patterns is associated with a significantly reduced cardiovascular disease risk, as well as the risk for other chronic diseases such as diabetes. In June 2006, the American Heart Association (AHA) released updated diet and lifestyle recommendations for preventing cardiovascular disease. The rec-

Table 1
Goals to Reduce Cardiovascular Disease Risk

☐ Consume an overall healthy diet

☐ Aim for recommended levels of low-density lipoprotein cholesterol, high-density lipoprotein cholesterol, and triglycerides

☐ Aim for a normal blood pressure

☐ Aim for a normal blood glucose level

☐ Be physically active

☐ Avoid use of and exposure to tobacco products

☐ Lose weight (avoid being overweight)

ommendations are summarized in the AHA tables 1 and 2.

FOLLOW A "HEART HEALTHY" DIET

The AHA recommends that people consume 25% to 35% of their total calories from fat, less than 7% of total calories from saturated fat, less than 1% of calories from trans fat, and less than 300 mg of cholesterol per day.

A diet that lowers LDL (the "bad" cholesterol) and raises HDL (the "good" cholesterol) is "heart healthy." Saturated fats and trans fats are major contributors to elevated LDL cholesterol. These fats both raise LDL, and trans fats also lower HDL cholesterol, thereby further increasing heart disease risk. The major source of saturated fat is animal fat (meat and dairy products) and the primary sources of trans fat are partially hydrogenated fats, used to prepare commercially fried and baked products. To limit your intake of these fats, choose leaner cuts of meats and choose skim or low-fat dairy products. Read nutrition labels and carefully avoid trans fat intake. (See Chapter 7.) The major contributors to low HDL cholesterol levels are elevated blood glucose, diabetes, elevated triglycerides, very low-fat diets (less than 15% of total calories from healthy fat sources), and excess body weight. An HDL cholesterol level below 40 mg/dL is a strong cardiovascular disease risk factor.

What is a normal glucose level? A normal blood glucose (sugar) level, when you have not eaten for at least eight hours, is below 100 mg/dL. When this level is 126 mg/dL or higher a person is diagnosed with diabetes. Type 2 diabetes is the most common type of diabetes, and obesity, especially abdominal obesity (excess belly fat), is a major risk factor for diabetes. Achieving even a modest weight loss (about 7% weight loss, which for a 150 pound person is about ten pounds) can delay and possibly prevent the onset of diabetes. Your doctor can determine your

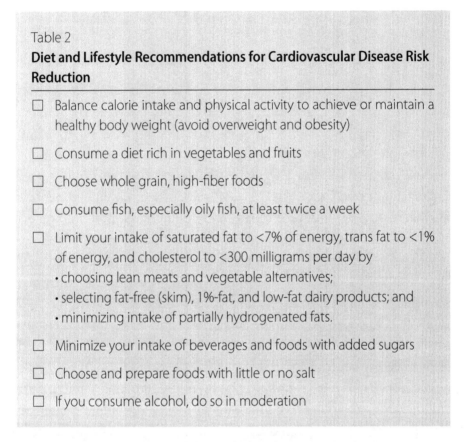

Table 2

Diet and Lifestyle Recommendations for Cardiovascular Disease Risk Reduction

☐ Balance calorie intake and physical activity to achieve or maintain a healthy body weight (avoid overweight and obesity)

☐ Consume a diet rich in vegetables and fruits

☐ Choose whole grain, high-fiber foods

☐ Consume fish, especially oily fish, at least twice a week

☐ Limit your intake of saturated fat to <7% of energy, trans fat to <1% of energy, and cholesterol to <300 milligrams per day by
• choosing lean meats and vegetable alternatives;
• selecting fat-free (skim), 1%-fat, and low-fat dairy products; and
• minimizing intake of partially hydrogenated fats.

☐ Minimize your intake of beverages and foods with added sugars

☐ Choose and prepare foods with little or no salt

☐ If you consume alcohol, do so in moderation

blood glucose level by means of blood tests.

Avoid all tobacco products. Smoking is a devastating risk factor for the development of heart disease. Studies also suggest that by giving up smoking your risk of dying from cardiovascular disease is lessened by more than 50% after only two years of quitting. It is that simple: quit smoking and give your heart the gift of longer life.

The AHA and the American College of Sports Medicine (ACSM) issued new guidelines on physical activity in 2007, updating the 1995 recommendations issued by ACSM and the CDC. The earlier recommendations stated that every U.S. adult should get 30 minutes or more of moderate intensity physical activity on most—preferably all—days of the week. The new guidelines recommend: Adults should get at least 150 minutes of moderate-intensity exercise per week. Exercise recommendations can be met through 30-60 minutes of moderate-intensity exercise (five days per week) or 20-60 minutes of vigorous-intensity exercise (three days per week). If you are older than 65, the new guidelines recommend that you also do strength training exercises (like lifting weights), and perform exercises that improve your balance and flexibility.

It is that simple: quit smoking and give your heart the gift of longer life.

It is true, eating more fruits and vegetables is good for you. Your parents were right. Diets rich in fruits and vegetables lower blood pressure and improve cardiovascular risk factors. Research studies show that people who eat a lot of fruits and vegetables have a lower risk of developing cardiovascular disease. An easy way to get the right variety is to choose fruits of many different colors, giving your body a wide range of valuable nutrients.

Eating whole-grain and high-fiber foods helps promote good health. Choose breads and cereals that list whole grains as the first item in the ingredient list over more highly processed grain products. There are simple ways to get more fiber in your diet:

- Choose whole-grain bread products
- Eat more fruits and vegetables
- Eat fruits and vegetables raw and leave the skin on
- Eat nuts (if not allergic).

You should also make fish a regular part of your diet. Research studies have found that regular fish consumption (1-2 meals/week) is associated with decreased deaths related to heart disease. This may be because fish and fish oils (omega-3 fatty acids) lower blood pressure and triglycerides. The evidence suggests that just two servings per week of fish that contain omega-3 fatty acid can lead to a 40% decrease in the likelihood of CHD death.

Because certain fish are contaminated with mercury and other organic compounds, consumers should check with local and state authorities and also check the FDA web site at www.fda.org for the most up-to-date information on recommendations for specific subgroups of the U.S. population (e.g., children and pregnant women) who should limit their fish intake.

As you can see, Frank was provided with a lot of information. "Are you ready to start making lifestyle changes now or are you still just 'thinking about it'?" his doctor asked. "I'm ready," Frank replied. He was then given an outline:

1. Write down your goals (both long-term and short-term).
2. Make a detailed plan. Write down what you will do each day to help accomplish your goals.
3. Consult your health care provider to ensure the safety and appropriateness of your plan.

> *Research studies have found that regular fish consumption (1-2 meals/week) is associated with decreased deaths related to heart disease.*

4. Line up support—family, friends, co-workers, and established community or commercial programs.
5. Follow your plan!
6. Continually revise and review your efforts to keep yourself on track.

Always remember: Be patient. Change may come gradually, but the benefits are worth it!

Frank was also encouraged to start with small, sustainable steps that he can begin to incorporate into his new lifestyle. For the first few weeks his doctor suggested that Frank try the following:

1. Park further from the front door of his workplace.
2. Take the stairs at work instead of the elevator.
3. Add one extra serving of vegetables to his dinner plate.
4. Bring a couple of pieces of fruit to work for a snack.
5. Avoid the vending machine snacks, which tend to contain high fat and high sugar.
6. Eat a good breakfast each morning.

Frank was now ready to go. With the help of his physician and family, he was on the way to making himself a new man.

Chapter 6

Prevent a Heart Attack: Reduce Your Stress

There it was! What hit Gloria Pitman as she walked into the conference room was an old familiar feeling, and it was becoming a habit. Like that, her heart was racing and she felt as if somebody had just punched her in the stomach. She had to remember to stay calm and take deep breaths. *I don't know how much more of this I can take,* she thought.

Dr. Pitman was not in a spot she would have chosen. Her whole career was at stake. It all depended on her keeping her wits about her. She was under an intense medical review because, allegedly, she did not follow the standard of care in the case of a patient who died of a heart attack under her care. Today was her meeting with the review board to go over the events and make their judgment. If Gloria was found guilty by this panel of her peers, she could no longer practice at the hospital she loved and had given her life to for so many years.

Gloria sat at one side of the long conference table. Looking at her from the other side was a wall of faces, all men, about to make their judgment on her. To make matters worse, when Gloria tried to make eye contact with one of the men across the room, he put his eyes down. Not a good sign.

Gloria was wound tighter than a dog on leash. She was afraid even to swallow, lest she give the impression that she was nervous. The panel was waiting to hear her version of the case. Then, in a voice that was both dry and gentle, she said: "Hello, I am Dr. Gloria Pitman."

Gloria had known plenty of stress in the past, but not like this. After her statement, while there was a short pause, Gloria kept reminding herself: "I am an excellent doctor with twenty years of experience. I survived my divorce. I put my daughter through college as a single mom. I survived my heart attack. Yes, I'm sick and tired, but I can get through this one too."

The worst part was the direct questioning about her medical judgment and the quality of care she gave. She wanted with all her will not to be defensive because she knew the facts would back her up. That was her tough side, but she was a vulnerable human being like all of us, so her voice was sometimes teary, and the tears said a lot. They said how angry she was, and how she had no way of expressing that anger.

Yes, her patient had died, despite the fact that she had done all she or any other cardiologist could. When she met with the family afterwards, she knew from their stony faces what the outcome would be: their eyes said she had killed their father, and she was pretty sure a review board would follow.

She had been jammed into the same box once before, and had been vindicated by the board, as she knew she would be this time too. But she still had to go through the ordeal, made worse this time by the presence of Dr. Ashland, whose questions were patronizing to her as an African-American woman.

"Dr. Pittman," he had asked, "I believe you were trained at, hmm, Morehouse Medical School." She wanted to say, "Yes, it was founded more than 35 years ago to address a serious problem: a shortage of African-American physicians. Its success has become legendary." Instead, she just said, "Yes."

Gloria's anger had a lot of roots, but most specifically in this scene she felt that she was reliving other similar ones she had been through, and they were not pretty scenes: she sensed that some of their questions showed bias against women. The questions also did not make an adjustment for her: they were loud, aggressive, and masculine. She was there as a scapegoat. Still, she had to answer the questions at face value because so much was on the line.

By now, Gloria was beginning to experience familiar symptoms, like shortness of breath, and she was a little sweaty. "May I take a break?" Dr. Ashland, the chairman of the board, said, "Of course. Dr. Pitman, are you all right?" Gloria nodded and Dr. Ashland went on: "We only have two more questions, and then we can all go home. But, okay, a fifteen minute break before we reconvene."

Gloria was not only a cardiologist, but she had also survived a heart attack. She knew that what she was feeling was the bad energy of stress, and she knew that stress was not good for her. So she made a vow to herself now that when this ordeal was over, she was going to slow down somehow. She just kept reminding herself that *while I can't always stop stressful events from happening, I can control the way I react to events, and not make the suffering worse.*

When Gloria returned to the conference room, she had been able to come to peace with the help of the reflection. She took comfort in knowing that no matter how this ended, she was going to be all right. She answered the last two questions from Dr. Ashland. Then she waited in another room as they convened. Dr. Ashland asked her to return to the conference room sooner than Gloria expected. She took a deep breath. "Dr. Pitman, we believe that you have acted in the best interests of the patient." With tears in her eyes, Gloria thanked the board and left.

STRESS MANAGEMENT

You already know why you must learn to manage stress. You must do it for your heart's sake and your life's sake, for those who love and need you and those you love and need. It is time now to learn some of the stress management techniques that have been proven effective by studies that have been going on for years.

Though we are speaking to you as an individual, our attempt is also to show you your place in the larger picture. We can start with the fact that these are not easy times. For a lot of people, and certainly for a great many African Americans, Latino Americans, and women, high degrees of stress are becoming the norm, and that is not good. From a social perspective, stress costs society a lot in terms both of the costs of an illness and the loss in productivity. It would seem the most obvious move would be to make stress-relief training free to us one and all. That would save so much money for everybody.

One way of coping is to know how to laugh. Believe it or not, laughter is strong medicine in the treatment of stress.

The core issue is human suffering—suffering that did not have to happen. Sad to say, there is no cure for stress that comes from outside conditions, like racism or just life itself. What we can do is to recognize the signs early and then, with methods we have learned by practice, breath a little healing into those stress signs.

So let us start thinking about it. When are you stressed, and under what circumstances? Start noticing. Write it down. Locate the pattern. Obviously, some of our most stressful moments happen when we are just minding our own business. It may be a red light that seems to have stayed on for a very long time, or something someone said to you. Sometimes, even innocent or trivial things can get to you. You are already handling all the stress you can carry, and one more thing takes you over the top. Keep a record of such and similar episodes in a stress diary.

When we get into these kinds of stresses, we are to some extent following a pattern. We have kind of lost our heads, and events already seem to have become uncontrollable, though we are hanging on by our fingertips.

One way of coping is to know how to laugh. Believe it or not, laughter is strong medicine in the treatment of stress. Our laughter already says out loud that we have found a new angle for looking at this crisis or semi-crisis or invented crisis. Sometimes, just putting on a smile can change your mood. Try it. It works.

We could talk all day about why and how laughter heals, and you will find many books on the subject in your library or bookstore. (Ask your librarian to recommend a title to you if you do not know exactly what you are looking for, just something on controlling stress.) Do not let yourself get into the very bad habit of never escaping stress, even when you are trying to have a good time, or just to sleep.

EXERCISE AS STRESS RELIEF

While we experience stress as a powerful negative emotion, one way of coping with it kills two birds with one stone. Nothing is better for the heart than regular exercise. Remember, the heart is a muscle and needs aerobic exercise.

The second benefit of exercise is that most people find even strenuous exercise relaxing. Ask anyone who regularly works out. They will tell you that even the stretching that is done at the beginning of the workout is calming. They breathe deeply and slowly, with each breath taking in a measure of greater tranquility. Just by deep steady breathing they are coming back to their bodies, and when our concentration is on the body, we can shut off the endless stream of thoughts that nag us.

Many of us have strong resistance to exercise and a long list of rationalizations for not doing it. We point to athletes who died running or playing sports. We remind ourselves of our aches and pains. How can anyone expect us to exercise when our body feels as miserable as it does? The reality is that most Americans get too little exercise, and more than two thirds of African-American men and an even higher percentage of women are not active enough to keep healthy.

Such inactivity leads to health problems. For example, roughly 40% of African-American women are overweight, and obesity is a risk factor for many illnesses, especially for heart disease. Extra weight often goes with higher cholesterol and increased risk of heart disease and even heart attack and stroke. It can also be a risk factor for high blood pressure and diabetes. Further, heart doctors find that older people who have remained active, even people in their seventies and eighties, live longer than inactive people thirty and forty years their juniors.

Some researchers have suggested that the reason African American women are more likely than white women to be obese is that black women burn fewer calories when they are at rest. Others, such as Shiriki Kumanyiki, professor of epidemiology at Penn State College of Medicine, as cited in the College of Health and Human Development's online magazine, attribute this difference to stress. Still others blame it on domestic arrangements (single mothers have no time to exercise) or socioeconomic factors (poor people cannot go to health clubs and the neighborhoods are not safe enough to allow jogging and other aerobic exercise). The fact is that many of America's, and the world's, greatest ath-

letes are African American—female athletes as well as male athletes. So it is obviously not impossible for African Americans to
be healthy and strong. Still, impossible or not, the data show that
black Americans do not exercise as much as whites, and that this
is one reason why heart disease and hypertension in the African-
American community are more common and, when incurred,
more severe. (Remember, the death rate from heart disease is
40 percent higher for black men and 70 percent higher for black
women than for their white counterparts.)

We recommend exercise for everyone who is capable of movement. Even bedridden patients can exercise, and nurses and physical therapists will be glad to provide instructions and assistance.
People who have had heart attacks will recover faster if they keep
to the levels of exercise their doctors recommend. People with
cardiovascular disease can improve their condition with a workout routine their doctor recommends. People who are perfectly
healthy also benefit. Healthy people can depend on their bodies
to take care of themselves only to a certain point. There comes
a time in everyone's life when we have to help the body to
help itself. It is the old adage: use it or lose it.

Some people help themselves by exercising with a friend so that they can strengthen each other's resolve.

It takes both patience and will power to start an exercise routine for the first time, and if you have not been physically active,
you will have to find ways to break through your resistance to exertion. Some people help themselves by exercising with a friend
so that they can strengthen resolve. If you have been a couch potato for a long time, you can start slowly. For example, walk to
the corner and back for a week. You will be delighted to find that
by the end of the week what was work to begin with has become
easy. Now start walking around the block. Do not let weather pre-

vent you. If you cannot walk outside, try the mall. If your neighborhood is not a good place for taking walks, go to one that is.

The first few weeks are the hardest. Most people find that after several weeks they no longer have to make much effort or will. Exercise soon becomes an important habit that they do not want to miss because exercise makes them feel good. Not only are feel-good hormones like endorphins released, but feeling fit and having stamina are powerful pay-offs in themselves. We know old people and some not so old who, if they miss exercise for a week, find they can hardly get out of a chair, but who, when exercising regularly, feel spry and vigorous.

Emotionally depressed people often find relief from exercise because it gets them out of the house, often in the company of others, as in a spa or Y or even in taking walks with companions. Regular exercise is a also a sure way to experience accomplishment, and success is good for the soul. Pay offs come easy. If you walk a quarter mile four or five days this week, you can walk half a mile next week or the week after. If you do arm exercises with fivepound weights this week, you will be eager to try the tens a few weeks later. Progress is built into exercise. All you have to do is to keep at it and soon you will find yourself growing stronger. There is no better medicine for depressed people than to discover that they not only can act, but they can also make progress. You begin to feel that if you can handle the weights or the aerobics, you can also handle the emotional weights you must lift to get through the day. (If you find that your feelings of depression do not go away, please see a doctor—you may have clinical depression, which is treatable with therapy and medication.)

Today, doctors recommend an hour of active exertion each day as the ideal program for keeping your heart healthy. Even three times a week can give you great benefits, and if you have only half an hour a day, that is far better than nothing. The time you spend in the gym is an investment. Your profit is a longer and happier life.

There is also plenty you can do between regular workout sessions. Walk instead of driving whenever you can. After a while you will begin to enjoy the chance it gives you to relax, breathe fresh air, see people, and simply feel the pleasure of having strong legs and good stamina.

Aerobic exercise, besides being perfect for your heart, is a better stress reliever than eating, smoking, drinking, or drugs. Each of the others involves cycles of dependency and craving. While taking your mind off the things you might be worried or angry about, exercise replaces negative feelings with a positive sense of well-being. So the greater the stress you are experiencing, the more important it is to exercise. Like meditation, exercise refreshes your mind, restores you, and helps you to face what had seemed overwhelming. So, let us review the core of the message. Moderate exercise may:

- Decrease blood pressure
- Raise good cholesterol (HDL)
- Lower bad cholesterol (LDL)
- Lower fat or triglyceride levels
- Help burn body fat
- Help relieve depression
- Build confidence and self-esteem
- Encourage you to make other lifestyle changes
- Provide, with proper diet, an effective means of controlling noninsulin diabetes
- Help relieve stress.

EXERCISE PRECAUTIONS

Obviously, there are precautions to keep in mind. If you have had heart problems or a heart attack, no matter what your age, talk to your doctor before you begin an exercise program to make sure that your heart can tolerate exercise. The same warning, of course, applies if you are recovering from bypass surgery, angioplasty, or stenting.

Those over forty who have not exercised in a long time also should consult their doctor before starting an exercise program. Of course, if you experience sudden shortness of breath or chest pains, stop exercising and get help. If it is extremely hot, avoid exercise outdoors or in a room that is not air-conditioned and avoid outdoor exercise if it is extremely cold. Do not exercise when you are ill with an extreme cold or flu, or if the air is bad, and do not exercise immediately after you eat, because it can cause cramps or nausea. Wait an hour or two, preferably two.

Keep in mind, too, that if you are beginning to exercise after a long layoff, you will need to build up slowly. Maybe you used to be able to swim seventy-six laps without breathing heavily. Now you are fifty and a little out of shape and can only swim two without stopping. Swim two. After you have done that three times for a week, you will feel ready to swim a lap or two more. That is the beauty of exercise. You get stronger and you can measure your progress. (Do not attempt to measure it at every session. Once a week is enough. That is when you can weigh yourself or gauge other progress.)

Maybe you once jogged five miles, but it has been a long time since you have walked more than three blocks. Start out with brisk walking. Feel your strength return. Before long, you may find yourself back to that five-mile jog. Moderation is the key.

Whatever exercise you are doing, spend a few minutes stretching and warming up before you begin. It will help you avoid injuries. By the same token, wear good, supporting shoes, comfortable clothing, and, if you are running or speed walking, avoid hard surfaces if at all possible. Many people jog in the streets these days, but if you are one of them, take reasonable care. It is easy to injure a foot or ankle on pavement.

Just as it is necessary to warm up, you also need to cool down when you have finished. That helps keep you from getting stiff and sore later. Cooling down is also beneficial because it allows your heart to return to its normal pace before you resume other activities. What this boils down to is that if you plan an hour of exercise, add fifteen minutes to it for warming up and cooling down.

GETTING STARTED

We are ready to go. You have set realistic goals for yourself, and you have vowed to make exercise a regular part of your routine, just like eating, showering, and sleeping. You are ready to tune in to your body. It will tell you if you are overdoing it; it will tell you when it is exhausted. Sometimes, when you are just starting, it will lie a little. Like you, it is out of practice, and the first time you break into a brisk walk, or try to pick up a light weight, it will start complaining. Learn to distinguish that resistance from real distress. In any case, once you have established your routine, the body stops resisting.

You will learn, after a while, that the weekly improvement you experience is all the competition you need.

Remember: You are not competing. When you first step into the gym, you may find yourself surrounded by a lot of people who are in better shape than you. They are not your concern. The simple trick about an exercise routine is that you begin where you are. If five-pound weights are all you can handle at the beginning, handle them. You will be amazed that in a few weeks the ten-pounders will feel just right. You will learn, after a while, that the weekly improvement you experience is all the competition you need. Even when you hit a plateau, the fact that you know you are healthier, and look better, and feel good, is quite enough.

Just as you need to be moderate in your goals, you can be moderate in your expenditure. These days, gyms can be fashion showcases. All you need is a shirt and shorts, a pair of gym shoes, and a pair of socks. Sure, you want the right shoes for what you are doing, but here too you can usually find bargains. Shop around. Do not spend a lot of money on exercise machines. If you belong to a gym, they will have machines. If you do not, there are plenty of exercises you can do with minimal or no equipment.

In most neighborhoods, there is a nearby community club or YMCA where you can work out regardless of your income. If you are broke and do not have a free gym available in a neighboring school or social center, you can get along fine by buying a few weights and an inexpensive book that tells you what to do with them. If the streets of your neighborhood are not fit for fast walking or jogging, go to a mall and walk around it three or four times. Or get on a bike or bus and go to a neighborhood that is safer.

When you are doing aerobic exercise—running, biking, swimming, or using a treadmill or stair climber—drink water to avoid dehydration. Use your mind along with your body. Many great athletes use mental imagery before they compete, fixing in their minds the actions they will soon be performing. You too, before you start your exercise, should take a few deep breaths and bring to mind the specific action you are about to perform. If you are getting ready to run or begin some other aerobic exercise, imagine your proud finish. You will find that such images can give you strength and courage, and can take your mind off the mere grinding aspect of exercise. It is a technique that works for champions. It can also work for you.

Early morning and late night are good times for exercise. These are times when you can find an hour or two for yourself— though admittedly, if you are a working parent (single or not), that may require getting up a bit earlier or going to sleep a bit later. In the morning, an exercise routine will energize you for the day. In the evening, it will relax you and help you unload tension. (Note: you may wish to avoid exercising just before bedtime. The stimulation may make it harder for you to fall asleep.)

Okay? Your goal is to burn 2,000 to 3,000 calories per week, at the rate of 300 to 500 calories per exercise period. Here is the menu:

CALORIE EXPENDITURE FOR ATHLETIC ACTIVITIES

These figures apply to a person weighing 150 pounds. Allow at 10 percent increase in caloric expenditure fore every 15 pounds over 150, and a 10 percent decrease for every 15 pounds under 150.

Activity	Calories Per Hour
Aerobic dancing	280-700
Backpacking	350-770
Badminton (competitive singles)	480
Basketball	360-600
Bicycling	
(10 mph)	420
(11 mph)	480
(12 mph)	600
(13 mph)	660

Calorie Expenditure for Athletic Activities, continued

Activity	Calories Per Hour
Calisthenics (heavy)	600
Gardening, lifting, stooping, digging	500
Golf (pull-carry clubs)	280–490
Handball	660
Hiking	660
Horseback riding	210–560
Mowing (push mower)	450
Rope skipping, vigorous	800
Rowing machine	840
Running	
(5 mph)	600
(6 mph)	750
(7 mph)	870
(8 mph)	1,020
(9 mph)	1,130
(10 mph)	1,235
Shoveling (heavy)	660
Skating, ice or roller, rapid	700
Skiing, downhill	600
Skiing, cross-country	
(2.5 mph)	560
(4 mph)	600
(5 mph)	700
(8 mph)	1,020
Snowshoeing	490–980
Swimming (25–50 yd/min)	360–750

Calorie Expenditure for Athletic Activities, continued

Activity	Calories Per Hour
Tennis, singles	420–480
Tennis, doubles	300–360
Walking, level road,	
4 mph (fast)	420
up stairs	600–1,080
up hill (3.5 mph)	480–900
Wood chopping	560

CALORIES BURNED ACCORDING TO WEIGHT PER HOUR

Activity	100 lbs.	150 lbs.	200 lbs.
Bicycling, 6 mph	160	240	312
Bicycling, 12 mph	270	410	534
Jogging, 7 mph	610	920	1,230
Jumping rope	500	750	1,000
Running, 5.5 mph	440	660	962
Running, 10 mph	850	1,280	1,664
Swimming, 25 yd/min	185	275	358
Swimming, 50 yd/min	325	425	650
Tennis, singles	265	400	535
Walking, 2 mph	160	240	312
Walking, 3 mph	210	320	416
Walking, 4.5 mph	295	440	572

OUR FINAL INSTRUCTIONS

How do you know when you are exercising at the proper rate? Check your pulse. You will have determined, with your doctor, the proper target rate. To find your pulse, the simplest method is to put your index and middle fingers on your radial artery, which you can feel pulsing just where the wrist merges with the forearm. Watching the second hand on a clock or your wrist-watch, count the number of times your pulse beats in fifteen seconds, and multiply by four.

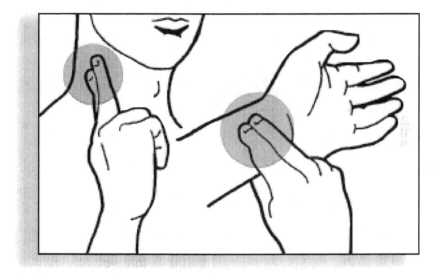

Check your heart rate by counting your pulse at the neck or wrist.

You can also take your pulse at the carotid artery in the neck by placing your index and middle fingers on the sternomastoid muscle. It is the one you feel when you turn your head to the side. Then count by the method described above. Do not press too hard. That can cause the heart to slow, or, if you have had carotid disease or a history of ministrokes, it may even cause a stroke. For that reason, check with your doctor before using this method—especially if you have diabetes or have had a stroke or previous brain damage.

Once again, a few warnings: Chest discomfort or tightness, or arm or neck pain during exercise could be signs of angina. Stop what you are doing and call for help or dial 911. Severe shortness of breath or excessive coughing while you are exercising also means you should stop. The same is true of bone or joint discomfort or severe muscle cramps or tendon soreness. Faintness, nausea, or vomiting during exercise means you should stop and see your doctor. The bottom line is to listen to your body and obey what it tells you.

Choose the form of exercise that feels most comfortable. Get your friends involved—take walks with them in the morning at a mall, a park, or a schoolyard. Walk to work or ride your bike if you can, and always walk rather than drive when the distances allow. Take a walk during your lunch break to a bookstore or to a place where you can eat lunch and rest your mind at the same time.

Choose the form of exercise that feels most comfortable.

Remember that aerobics do not necessarily mean running, nor do they require equipment. Fast walking or power walking are excellent exercises, giving most of the benefits of running, but avoiding the risks of injury. If you want to stay indoors, your own staircase is an excellent conditioner. Just walk up and down carefully and at your own pace. If you are elderly, you may wish to do this exercise in the company of a loved one or a friend who can help you if help is needed.

If you like to exercise to music, step classes are fun. They are available at the YMCA or your local health club. You can also do them at home with the help of a TV set and a 4-6″ lift as equipment.

And do not ignore resistance exercises. Even if you do not want to be Superman or Superwoman, training with free weights or weight machines, just like aerobic exercise, improves your cholesterol profile, helps control your weight, and helps control conditions such as diabetes. Because such exercises also enhance flexibility and balance, they help you live with degenerative diseases such as arthritis. Weight training is not reserved for men. Because women often suffer muscle atrophy, it is also most beneficial to them.

In working with weights, especially free weights, have an instructor nearby, especially when you begin. Remember that it is far better to go for multiple repetitions at a comfortable weight than to try to impress people by pushing weights far too heavy for you. Your aim is to improve your muscle tone and strength, but not, as power lifters do, to go for bulk.

The world is your gym. You do not need riches or power to join. Your own body, just as it is, is the only ticket required for admission.

Before we close this part of the discussion, we want to say a few words about exercising when you suffer from a disease that weakens you or in some other way prevents you from performing fully. Arthritis is one such disease. A degenerative joint disease, it is often associated with pain, and those who suffer from it cannot handle weights without making that pain worse. For them, the most popular exercise is swimming. Bicycling is also a good sport for sufferers from arthritis, unless knee pain prevents it.

Patients with diabetes can also benefit from exercise. It helps lower the blood sugar, and in some cases even allows the patient to go off medication or insulin. Walking is an excellent exercise for diabetics. Remember that the appropriate footwear is important to help protect the feet and legs from injury caused by the poor blood flow that accompanies diabetes.

Patients recovering from heart surgery or a heart attack will do supervised exercise as part of their cardiac rehab program. Once that is done, with their doctor's approval, they will return to normal life—which means normal exercise.

Finally, if your cholesterol or triglyceride levels are abnormally high, exercise may help to decrease bad cholesterol (LDL) and triglyceride levels. Aerobic exercise increases good cholesterol.

AVOID ISOLATION

Suffering stress in isolation can feel like torture. Ironically, chronic stress often leads to isolation; it involves self-obsession, depression, and feelings of worthlessness. Sometimes, stressed and depressed people, angry and even disgusted with themselves, also act hostilely toward others, taking their misery out on whoever is at hand. Naturally, under such conditions, you may find yourself pulling away from family and friends.

Remember that we are social animals, not made to live in isolation. If you feel cut off from friends and family, go to a park where there are children. Watch them play. Listen to them laugh. Their laughter will awaken something in you with which you may have fallen out of touch.

Sure, people get busy and forgetful, but most of us are delighted when we get a call from someone who wants to see us.

Doing errands can help. They require you to leave the house, go somewhere, and interact with people, if only on a formal level. The bottom line is that you are making human contact, and human contact often involves laughter and kindness.

When you are depressed, you sit around waiting for people to call you, and when they do not, that becomes just more proof that you are no good and no one loves you any more than you love yourself. Try making a call or two. The first call is the hardest. Sure, people get busy and forgetful, but most of us are delighted when we get a call from someone who wants to see us. Have lunch with a friend, or arrange an evening get-together with several friends. It may feel hard to do, but it is a way of acting, doing something for you, breaking the terrible passive resignation that stress imposes. Give and take with others pulls us back out of brooding and into the sun. So find someone to talk to. Often, what others can offer is not advice, just a kind listening ear, and that can be just the medicine a stressed person needs.

STRESS ON THE JOB

A certain amount of job stress may be unavoidable. Repetitive work, especially under a bullying (or, sometimes, sexist or racist) boss can be a true nightmare from which you can escape only by seeking a new job or even learning new skills.

Insofar as the job allows, you often can improve things for yourself. For most people, what causes stress on the job is the feeling of powerlessness. Where possible, then, be an active citizen in the workplace. Ask questions and make suggestions. Cultivate good relationships with fellow workers. Sometimes that sense of solidarity can be the beginning of a renewed sense of control.

Experts urge you to be decisive and assertive at work. "How do I get there from here?" you may ask. Simply writing down what the problem is and a list of your options for solving it—even the option of doing nothing—can be an excellent start. List not only the obvious solutions but also the unusual ones; and for each, list their pros and cons. Sometimes, through such a process, you discover that problems that seemed to have no solu-

Get into the habit of saying what you think, knowing what you want, and doing what is in your power to get it.

tions actually have several. Play with those solutions. Be flexible, keeping in mind that if you decide on one and it does not pay off, you can turn to another. The mere activity of working toward a solution will bring its own rewards. Action, in such matters, is nearly always preferable to inaction, and clear and patient thought can be a form of action.

SLEEP

Certainly if you are sleepless because of stress, you need to correct the problem. Sleeplessness feeds stress and makes you moody, angry, more vulnerable to illness, and to the things that caused you stress in the first place. Regulating your sleep should be a top priority.

That means avoiding stimulants like alcohol, caffeine, and nicotine. All of them can disrupt sleep. Develop good habits for getting ready to sleep. If you watch a violent movie before going to bed, you are not likely to slip easily into sleep. Find ways to calm yourself before bed. Read something that soothes or even bores you. Listen to mellow music. Once in bed, remove the obvious obstacles to sleep. Use ear plugs to eliminate annoying noise. Relax your body by methodically tensing and then relaxing muscles—first your feet, then gradually up your legs, the trunk of your body, your chest, neck, jaw, cheeks, and brow. Do it a few times if necessary. It works.

Giving attention to your breathing can also help. Try to steady and slow it. Give your attention to your breath. When your mind wanders, bring it back, gently, to the breath.

If none of this helps, other resources are available. Ask your doctor to refer you to a sleep clinic where you can get medical treatment or treatment through biofeedback. We do not recommend over-the-counter sleep enhancers. If you are suffering sleep problems, self-medication can be risky. It is best to talk to your doctor.

PRAYER AND MEDITATION

For some people, turning the mind to something or someone larger than the self is an effective way of coping with stress. The cardiologist Dr. Randolph Byrd reports that patients who pray daily are less likely to be sick than those who do not pray and, if they become sick, the sickness will be less severe. While prayer may play a major role in the lives of some cardiovascular patients, it should not replace seeking medical care, going to the doctor, and adhering to the treatment plan prescribed.

Another spiritual discipline for managing stress is meditation. Many people have found in meditation a practical exercise that calms them and allows them to taste life's fruits more fully. These days, in major cities, meditation centers are easy to find, and many of them offer free or inexpensive instruction. The basic principles of meditation are simple enough, and you can begin them without instruction.

Pick a time of day and a place reasonably quiet and free from distractions and interruptions. Sit on a thick cushion on the floor, legs crossed, or in a straight-backed chair, keeping an upright posture so that your back is not supported by the back of the chair. Your spine, your neck, and the top of your head should all be in a line, as though someone were pulling you up with a string attached to the top of your head. In other words, sit tall.

Sit still, resting your hands palms down on your thighs. Rest your eyes also, using a soft gaze, on a point about five feet ahead of you on the floor. Keep your gaze there but gently, without fixing your focus. Locate your breathing in your abdomen. You can do this by pushing your breath all the way out on the exhale and then sending your awareness to the in-and-out taking of your breath. Do this for 10 or so breaths, until you've located your breathing. Then just breathe naturally, without trying to breathe in any special way, but being aware of your breathing as it goes in and out of its own accord.

These days, in major cities, meditation centers are easy to find, and many of them offer free or inexpensive instruction.

You might begin by sitting for 10 minutes a day, or 10 minutes twice a day, and then lengthen the time as you get used to the practice. Set a timer so that you do not need to watch the clock. It is more important to maintain a continuity of practice from day to day than to sit for longer periods of time. For example, sit for 10 minutes every day when you get up rather than sitting for 30 minutes on Monday and then not getting back to it until Thursday.

You will notice as you sit that your mind produces an endless stream of images, worries, plans, daydreams, and thoughts, both positive and negative. They race in, one after another. At the beginning stage, the steady urgency with which your mind spins out these random thoughts can be shocking and disagreeable. This is what the Buddhist's call "monkey mind" or "grasshopper mind"—for obvious reasons. Meditation trains the mind to regard this endless stream as a passing show, with no one thought being more important than another. When you find yourself getting caught up in your plans for the day, a pressing appointment, anxiety about your children, meal plans, vacation plans, or fantasies, just label this "thinking" and return your awareness to your breathing and to the present moment.

The point is to stay alert and relaxed, letting thoughts come and go. When you catch yourself getting caught up in one of them, simply label it "thinking," and return to your breathing. This will happen over and over in the course of 10 minutes. Just keep starting over, going back to the breathing and bringing yourself back to the present. Meditation is sometimes falsely looked at as a way to "clear your mind." You will not clear it, but you will learn to regard it in a different way—with equanimity.

PROFESSIONAL THERAPY

Much of what we have been talking about has to do with combating stress through our own efforts. Sometimes our problems become more than we can handle alone. That is when, blessedly, we can turn to professional institutions and people to help us. For example, we highly recommend twelve-step programs such as Alcoholics Anonymous and similar programs designed to help us kick bad habits and heal us of the shame that helped plunge us into the dependency in the first place. In a support group you can share your most painful feelings of shame, guilt, and stress without losing face. Listening to the moving and sometimes heroic stories of others helps put our own situation in perspective.

These days, support groups are available to almost everyone. Many people have found that being in a protected space where they can laugh freely, and cry, is in itself good medicine. It is also, for people who have allowed shame and powerlessness to isolate them, the beginning of a return to the social world.

Finally, when all else fails, there is therapy. Your doctor or your minister should be able to refer you to a counselor who can provide the help you need. Sometimes a few sessions do the job, by shifting our focus that half inch necessary to bring us back to positive life. Sometimes it takes longer. Sometimes the counseling is sufficient. Sometimes it is necessary to get a prescription for one of the many effective antidepressants or stress relievers available these days. Therapy is there for you. It is a tool for your benefit. Do not hesitate to use it to your advantage.

Our basic theme is simple, and we will repeat it one more time to be sure that it is clear: No one has to be driven over the edge of despair by stress. Resources are available to help you find your way back to a productive and loving

Many people have found that being in a protected space where they can laugh freely, and cry, is in itself good medicine.

life. Have pride and courage and choose to live.

CHANGING YOUR THOUGHTS

One of the ways that people can be lazy is by not changing their minds. It is easier, or seems to be, to keep on in our old ways, which are familiar and give our lives the appearance of comfortable routine. The only trouble is that we ourselves, the people we know, and the world itself are constantly changing around us, and if we get into some private lockstep, we may start feeling that we are being knocked around simply because we are out of synch with the way life actually works. People do not act as we think they should, the mainstream news is worse than it ought to be, you find that you cannot pay your bills, you get ill, a friend falls away from you, a loved one dies. These things "shouldn't" happen, but they do.

Often, we just have to ride out the storm. Fighting it is useless. Many aspects of our lives are not within our power to control. These are the ones we must learn to live with if we are to avoid unnecessary stress.

Naturally, we suffer when bad things happen. But we still have the freedom not to add to our suffering by resisting or denying what has already happened. Eventually, we all must make peace with even the bitterest blows. The alternative is endless misery. When we speak of stress relief, we are talking about making that peace.

For some people prayer, meditation, exercise, being with others, laughter, and taking deep breaths are ways of "changing our thoughts" and putting distance between ourselves and our grief. Of course suffering is real, and we all get through it the best we can. The trick is not to make it worse. We can grieve, mourn, pay all necessary homage to disasters and setbacks, but in the end we need to find a way to get on with our lives.

Even people who feel as if they have always been run by convictions and emotions as unchangeable as the rising of the sun can, by doing the things that make them feel better in body and soul, recover from grief, turn their lives around after disaster, and come back stronger than before, because loss and grief can be powerful teachers. Think of it this way, you always have enough strength to open the next door. It just takes patience, determination, and right choices. Learning to manage stress is among the greatest gifts you can give yourself. Many others have done it, and you can too.

Eventually, we all must make peace with even the bitterest blows. The alternative is endless misery.

Here is the formula: know what you want and be sure that what you want is not unrealistic. To be healthy in body and soul and to maintain cardiovascular wellness is realistic for many people. It is an obtainable goal. In doing so, one can honor the gift of life given to us as we attempt to make our time on earth as fruitful and pleasant as it is in our power to make it.

Chapter 7

Choosing What to Eat

W E STILL LOVE THE MEALS passed down from our ancestors. Today we know that for our hearts' sakes we must cut down not only on calorie intake but on our consumption of saturated fats, cholesterol, and sodium as well. We must also increase our intake of fruits and vegetables, whole grains, and, in the place of butter and lard, monounsaturated fats.

Here is a rough estimate of what we need:

- 1,600 calories for most women and older adults
- 2,200 calories for kids, teenage girls, active women, and most men
- 2,800 calories for teenage boys and active men

Most foods contain several types of fat. Saturated fats are found in animal products such as meat, whole milk and other dairy products, and lard. Certain vegetable oils, like palm, palm kernel, coconut oils, and cocoa butter are sources of saturated fats. This latter group is sometimes referred to as tropical fats. Tropical fats, though heavily saturated, do not contain cholesterol. Like all saturated fats, they raise blood cholesterol.

That is what saturated fats do: While they may not themselves contain cholesterol, they raise the cholesterol in the blood. A food like potato chips can be "cholesterol-free" but still very high in saturated fats. Keep in mind that the now common marketing ploy that a food is cholesterol-free may simply mean that you need to take a closer look at the nutritional label.

Despite the danger that fats can pose to the body, the body needs fat. It is a good energy source, it promotes a healthy nervous system, and it protects against mental decline. That need is best satisfied with monounsaturated fats. Instead of raising your bad cholesterol level, they actually lower it. In addition, they increase your good cholesterol.

Olive oil is an excellent source, as are peanut oil and canola oil. That is why we recommend that you use them as much as possible in your cooking, rather than saturated fats. Monounsaturated fats are often found in many fish and seafood (mackerel and salmon are especially good sources), and also in nuts, olives, and avocados.

Keep in mind that the now common marketing ploy that a food is cholesterol-free may simply mean that you need to take a closer look at the nutritional label.

Polyunsaturated fats are found in safflower, sunflower, corn, soybean, cottonseed, and sesame oils. They too are effective as cholesterol busters, as they lower bad cholesterol.

If you want a physical image to guide you, think of it this way. The more solid a fat is at room temperature, the more saturated it is. Lard and shortening are very solid and therefore very saturated. Stick margarine and butter are still pretty solid and are very saturated. Tub margarine and butters are better, oils are better still, and cooking sprays are best.

Now consider omega-3 fatty acids. These are found in fish and fish oils and in canola oil. Canola oil is so effective in lowering blood cholesterol as well as triglyceride levels that we recommend it even above olive oil. (Omega-3 fatty acids are also found in soybeans, certain nuts and seeds.)

You can buy fish oils in health food stores, but a better and cheaper source is a frequent diet of fish and shellfish (at least once or twice a week). Remember that even the fattiest fish— salmon—is far leaner than the leanest beef. That is true also of shrimp, scallops, lobster, etc. Some people avoid them because of their cholesterol content. The good they will do with their fatty acids far outweighs the cholesterol they contain. (Just go easy on the butter and tartar sauce.)

If you put your reading glasses on and go down the list of ingredients in processed or snack food you have in the cupboard, you will run into another oil, usually called partially hydrogenated vegetable oil. Now that you know it, limit your use of it. Though it begins as a safe vegetable oil, it is hydrogenated so that the product can sit long on the shelf, and the hydrogenation process makes it become very saturated. These fats, also known as trans-fatty acids, not only cause cholesterol to increase but they may pose a risk for certain types of cancers.

Eating the right kind of fat can lower your risks of coronary artery disease and heart attack. Fat is fat, and it means calories. If we eat more calories than we burn off, the extra calories are stored as body fat, no matter from where those calories are derived. People know this, presumably, and that is why we have seen so many fat-free products in the grocery markets. Unfortunately, they do not seem to do much good. While they have helped Americans cut their fat intake from 36 percent to 34 percent of their average daily calories, during the same period we have gained 8 pounds per person!

The problems may be that fat-free foods, whether as meals or snacks, do not fill us as fatty foods do. So we end up eating more of them, and in the process, we take in more calories. Do not fall into the illusion that because a food is fat-free you can eat all you want. That could be a heavy mistake.

Another fad has been fat substitutes that deliver some of the desirable qualities of fat, but add fewer calories. Some of them—cellulose gel Avicel, guar gum, and gum Arabic—have been around for a long time and are considered safe. There are a number of other fat substitutes on the market, the best known being Olestra. Some of them are still high in saturated fats and high in calories. We recommend you use these substitutes sparingly and with some caution.

SODIUM

Time for everything you always wanted to know about salt. The main thing you know already: If you have high blood pressure or if you are salt-sensitive, you need to follow a low-salt diet—2,000 to 3,000 milligrams a day—because salt can make hypertension worse. For the rest of us, a "no added salt" diet works fine. It allows from 3,000 to 4,000 milligrams a day, which is a liberal allowance.

While most of us have not given much thought to whether we are salt-sensitive, African Americans tend to be more so than Caucasian Americans. So, playing the odds, and given the very high rate of hypertension among African Americans, you are probably doing yourself a favor to cut back on salt, if you do not cut it out altogether.

That is actually easier to do than you might think. The taste for salt is learned, which means that it can be unlearned. Within two months of not adding salt to your food, your taste buds will have become so sensitized that salted foods will taste oversalted. At that point, you will find that your tongue is taking in all kinds of new taste pleasures that previously were masked by salt.

The hard part about reducing salt is that many prepared foods contain sodium, although you may not think of them as especially salty. A half cup of chocolate-flavored instant pudding, for example, has 470 milligrams of sodium, and two slices of bacon have 245 milligrams. Cheese, cured meats, canned soups, commercial tomato sauce, many snack and fast foods, foods that contain monosodium glutamate (common in Chinese food), and baked foods with baking soda and baking powder are all high in sodium.

While most of us have not given much thought to whether we are salt-sensitive, African Americans tend to be more so than Caucasian Americans.

We recommend that you make your own dishes. That way, you are within your power to feed yourself and your family what is good for all of you and to control the salt. If, after a while on a no-salt-added diet, you still have a craving, you can afford the occasional luxury of salted nuts or chips. You may find that you do not need salt at all. Using herbs and spices will give your food a new kind of zest that you and your family may in the end find tastier than salt.

FIBER

Another nutritional gift you can give your heart is fiber. (To call fiber "nutritional" is a little misleading, because not all fiber is digested. Unsoluble fiber passes through the intestines, drawing water with it, and is eliminated.) High-fiber diets lower cholesterol. One study shows that among two groups of people on a reduced-fat diet, those who took 25 grams of fiber a day lowered their cholesterol by 13 percent; those who did not, lowered their cholesterol by only 9 percent. It is not known why fiber lowers cholesterol. One theory suggests that it may bind to cholesterol and bile acids in the intestines and prevent the body from absorbing them, so they are excreted with other body wastes.

Because fiber seems to work that way, and because, in addition, it helps prevent colon cancer and other intestinal problems (pectin, a kind of fiber found in apples, grapefruits, and oranges, may specifically protect against heart disease), it is important that you take in 20 to 35 grams daily. Soluble fiber is found in oat bran, beans and other legumes, barley, prunes, and various fruits and vegetables. If you do not keep up your diet with such foods, you can get fiber in the form of psyllium, a natural grain grown in India and found commercially as Metamucil, Fiberall, and Perdiem.

Another nutritional gift you can give your heart is fiber.

Because fiber draws water from the body, it is important that you increase your water intake as you increase your fiber intake. It is also true that diets high in fiber can cause bloating and gas. Usually, that problem vanishes once you have made fiber a regular part of your diet. If you are having trouble with gas, this can be relieved by an enzyme marketed as Beano, which is sold over the counter. If beans—one good source of fiber—are the cause of the problem, add 1/8 teaspoon of baking soda to the water in which you soak the beans.

VITAMINS

Vitamins, whether you get them as part of a good and varied diet, or as supplements purchased at the drug store, are important to the health of your heart. Your doctor can tell you whether he thinks you should take vitamin supplements.

NUTRITION AND THE GROCERY STORE

Now that we have established some general principles of nutrition, let us go shopping. The produce and dairy foods are simple. You will want to pick up lots of fruits, vegetables, whole grains, and low-fat, low-cholesterol dairy products.

Now comes the hard part: How do you know what you are getting when you buy packaged and prepared foods?

Here are some important things to know about the list of ingredients that appears on all packaged food.

- The most helpful parts of the label are the *ingredient list* and the *nutrition facts*.
- Ingredients are listed in order of the amount used, from the most to the least.
- The types of fat—saturated, monounsaturated, or polyunsaturated—and their order on the list is important. Check them. Manufacturers often use two or more types of fat and list them separately farther down the list than they would be if they were grouped together. In that case, fat may not appear to be a major ingredient when it is. Check this.
- Claims that a product contains no cholesterol are misleading. A product free of cholesterol may be very high in fat—even saturated fat! Check this on the list.
- Some products, acceptable in small portions, contribute too much fat to the diet if eaten in large quantities. Check the portion size on the nutritional label.

Before leaving home, make a shopping list that includes enough of the basic and staple foods to last until your next planned trip to the store.

Done shopping? We know it took a little longer because you

had to read all those labels. Next time it will go faster. Anyway, now you are home and it is time to start thinking about cooking and eating.

Because you are now into low-fat cooking, you will have to make some adjustments. Fat serves several functions: It adds moisture, it carries or enhances flavor, it gives food a certain feel in your mouth, and it makes you feel full. As you make the transition to low-fat cooking, an adjustment you will need to make so that you and your family will not feel taste deprived is to spark your cooking with new herbs and spices.

WHAT THE LABELS MEAN

Label Claim	Definition
Calorie-free	Less than 5 calories
Low calorie	40 calories or less
Light or lite	1/3 fewer calories or 50 percent less fat than the standard product. If more than half the calories are fat, the fat content must be reduced by 50 percent or more.
Light in sodium	50 percent less sodium than the standard product
Fat-free	Less than 1/2 gram fat
Low fat	3 grams or less fat
Cholesterol-free	Less than 2 milligrams cholesterol and 2 grams or less saturated fat
Low cholesterol	20 milligrams or less cholesterol and 2 grams or less saturated fat
Sodium-free	Less than 5 milligrams sodium
Very low sodium	35 milligrams sodium
Low sodium	140 milligrams or less sodium
High fiber	5 grams or more fiber

Food label guide

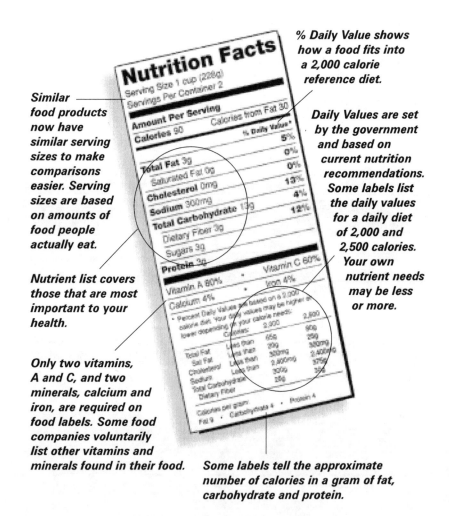

Similar food products now have similar serving sizes to make comparisons easier. Serving sizes are based on amounts of food people actually eat.

Nutrient list covers those that are most important to your health.

Only two vitamins, A and C, and two minerals, calcium and iron, are required on food labels. Some food companies voluntarily list other vitamins and minerals found in their food.

% Daily Value shows how a food fits into a 2,000 calorie reference diet.

Daily Values are set by the government and based on current nutrition recommendations. Some labels list the daily values for a daily diet of 2,000 and 2,500 calories. Your own nutrient needs may be less or more.

Some labels tell the approximate number of calories in a gram of fat, carbohydrate and protein.

Note: Numbers on nutrition labels may be rounded.

Many herbs and spices are said to be good for you. They also taste terrific. Try them out to see which of them, and which combinations, best please your palate. Just to give you an idea of the range, there is freshly grated ginger, garlic, citrus zest, dry mustard, hot peppers, dried fruits, and dried vegetables like tomatoes that will color and intensify your cooking in ways you never imagined. You will also find a number of salt-free blends on the spice shelves.

As for the recipes themselves, there is no need to abandon the old ones, although you will probably want to add some new ones to mark your new cooking style. Most recipes can easily be adapted to lower-fat versions simply by substituting ingredients that are high in total fat, saturated fat, or cholesterol with lower-fat alternatives. Sometimes an ingredient will have to be eliminated altogether because no low-fat alternative is available, or you can just reduce the amount of that high-fat ingredient.

Just remember that, while you are learning this new style, you will need to examine each ingredient carefully so that, at each step of your recipe, you can cut the fat. It may be as easy as frying in a nonstick skillet with a spritz of vegetable spray instead of adding globs of butter or oils. Or you may wish to substitute ground turkey for ground beef. The turkey has 50 percent less saturated fat than other ground meats!

Here is a list of substitutions you can make when you are cooking—and some that work even when you are eating out.

LIST OF SUBSTITUTIONS

Instead of	Use
1 tbsp. butter	1 tsp. margarine or 1/4 tbsp. canola, peanut, or olive oil
1 cup butter	3/4 cup canola or olive oil
1 cup shortening	2/3 cup canola or olive oil
1 whole egg	2 egg whites or 1/4 egg substitute
1 cup sour cream	1 cup low-fat yogurt (plain) whole milk skim or 1 percent milk
1 cup cream	evaporated skim milk or evaporated milk
whipped cream or topping containing saturated fat	pressurized whipped cream (2 tbsp. = 1 gram fat, 16 calories)
mayonnaise	light mayonnaise
ice cream	low-fat frozen yogurt, ice milk, sorbet, ices, etc.
1 oz. baking chocolate	3 tbsp. baking cocoa plus 1 tbsp. oil
cottage cheese	low-fat cottage cheese (but be aware that "low-fat cottage cheese still contains 4% milk-fat)
bacon, sausage, hot dogs	Canadian bacon or lean ham
beef	lean ground round, ground sirloin, turkey or chicken (10 percent fat)
cheese	low-fat cheese (2 to 6 grams fat/oz.)
salad dressing	low-calorie salad dressing
1 can cream soup	homemade white sauce: 1 cup skim milk, 1 tbsp. margarine, 2 tbsp. flour
canned spaghetti sauce	6 oz. tomato paste and 18 oz. water to 1 jar of sauce

potato chips on casseroles	bread crumbs or cereal crumbs (for example, corn flakes)
cakes, cookies, brownies	vanilla wafers, gingersnaps, crackers, fortune cookies, angel food cake, fruit
sausage/pepperoni pizza	vegetarian pizza
packaged lunch meats	thinly sliced deli meats—chicken, beef
croissants	bagels, English muffins, soft pretzels
french fries	homemade oven fries (no more than 1 tsp. oil/ serving
chips	popcorn, pretzels
2-crust pies	one-crust or graham cracker crust

ADDITIONAL COOKING AND DINING TIPS

- Use a minimum amount of fat in cooking.
- Avoid frying and deep-fat frying. Use low-fat cooking methods—bake, broil, microwave, steam, poach, grill.
- Trim fat from meat before and after cooking.
- Remove poultry skin.
- Tenderize lean cuts of meat with marinades, mechanical pounding, or a tenderizer.
- Cook longer at low heat rather than shorter at high heat.
- Use moist heat, adding liquid or using meat's own juices, where appropriate.
- Remove fat from soups and stews by making them a day early, then refrigerating and skimming solid fat.
- Drain all fat from cooked ground beef. Pat with pa-

per towels and wipe out the pan before adding spices, vegetables, etc.

- Make pasta, legumes, rice, or vegetables the focus of the meal instead of meat.
- Use smaller portions of meat, fish, and poultry.
- Include meatless meals using beans and legumes.
- Use nonstick pans or sprays.
- Invest in a sharp knife to remove fat from meat and poultry and to cut thin slices for stir-fry dishes.
- Use nonfat dry milk and skim milk in cooking soups, puddings, casseroles, and muffins.
- Use cheese as a garnish. Sprinkle small amounts on top of casseroles, etc.
- Use herbs, spices, and butter alternatives to flavor vegetables, soups, etc.

Chapter 8

Effects of
Overweight and Obesity
on Heart Disease

Despite all of the latest medical knowledge and advances in cardiovascular health treatments, a major risk factor for heart disease is being overlooked—being overweight. Most Americans, regardless of sex, age, gender, race, economic status, or education, eat too much. Period. Despite all of the press on losing weight, the problem continues to rapidly grow. Simply stated, being overweight is just plain horrible for your heart and overall cardiovascular health.

The prevalence of those who are overweight and obese in the United States has risen to epidemic proportions. Obesity and being overweight are major medical problems affecting adults and children alike. According to the World Health Organization, in 2005 1.6 billion adults were overweight (BMI>25kg/m2) and 400 million people were obese (BMI>30kg/m2). It is projected that by 2015 about 2.3 billion adults will be overweight and over 700 million will be obese.

Today, nearly 70 percent of adult people are classified as overweight or obese, compared to the 1980s and 1990s, where 50 percent of adults were obese. It has been extensively documented that this medical problem (overweight and obesity) is associated with greater morbidity than poverty, alcoholism and smoking. Furthermore, there is new evidence that obesity could soon outpace cigarette abuse as the leading cause of preventable mortality in the U.S.

Traditional treatments to achieve healthy weight loss such as diets, lifestyle changes, and behavioral therapy have not worked and the consequences have further caused overweight and obesity to be independent risk factors of poor cardiovascular health, greatly impacting long term survival.

Obese people, in fact, have a 75% greater risk of death from any cause than normal weight people.

SCOPE OF MEDICAL PROBLEMS ASSOCIATED WITH OBESITY AND BEING OVERWEIGHT

It has been extensively documented that obesity and being overweight adversely effects cardiovascular health and exacerbates chronic disease states. The adverse effects of obesity are as follows:

- **Insulin Resistance.** Obesity increases insulin resistance, glucose intolerance and can lead to metabolic syndrome (briefly defined as hypertension, type 2 diabetes, and abnormal lipids).
- **Hypertension and abnormal lipid levels.** Hypertension (high blood pressure) and abnormal lipid levels are associated with obesity. Total cholesterol, Triglycerides, LDL, non HDL, and small dense LDL, are all increased, and HDL and apolipoprotein-A1 are all decreased.

Obesity, structurally and functionally, adversely affects the heart

Obesity can lead to remodeling of the heart, causing overall heart dysfunction. Also, heart failure, coronary artery disease, atrial fibrillation, and left atrial enlargement are associated with obesity and being overweight. Obesity is also associated with pulmonary hypertension, obstructive sleep apnea and sleep disordered breathing, all of which are known to negatively impact heart health. The main point here is that being overweight is really bad for your heart.

Obesity, Overweight and Obesity Cardiomyopathy

Obesity cardiomyopathy is defined as heart disease that is not secondary to hypertension, type 2 diabetes, coronary artery disease, or other causes. Obesity and overweight are now considered to be independent risk factors for CVD and heart failure, and are the major causative factors in obesity cardiomyopathy. Also, it is important to know that obesity cardiomyopathy is often under-recognized and under diagnosed, especially in overweight or obese patients who do not have diabetes, hypertension, coronary disease or dyslipidemia. Finally, because this disease is not well studied, obese patients with heart failure are usually treated with conventional medication, including Beta blockers, which could be harmful in obese patients.

Obesity and Stroke

There are multiple studies showing that as one's BMI increases, even by 1Unit, the risk of ischemic stroke increase by 4%. The etiology for this could be due to hypertension, atrial fibrillation, or a prothrombotic state often seen in the obese.

Obesity and sudden cardiac death

Sudden cardiac death, secondary to ventricular arrhythmias, has been reported in patients with obesity cardiomyopathy. The reasons for this are not clear but may be associated with increased electrical irritability of the heart, or fatty infiltrates around the heart's conduction system often present in obese and overweight patients.

As stated previously and here for emphasis, overweight and obesity are independent risk factors for cardiovascular health and can alone adversely affect cardiovascular health. Being overweight is bad for your heart, period. It is also a major problem for millions of people who have tried losing weight for years, only to fail. We believe that eating healthy and exercising should always, as has been stressed in previous chapters, be a way of life; but the fact is, it simply is not how the majority of us are living.

Real solutions for obesity and overweight

There are hundreds of ways to lose weight, evidenced by the trillion-dollar weight loss industry. There are methods that seem to work for certain individuals and not for others. Often, individuals lose weight, just to gain it back again, and then some. Diets, restrictive diets, have been proven to be not effective for long-term weight loss. The bottom line is, for you to lose weight, you need to change your behaviors, and that is a major milestone for anyone.

To lose weight you need to consume fewer calories than you burn off in a given day. This can be done by consuming fewer calories, or exercising more, or both. For the morbidly obese, there are surgeries that can aid in this process, although the patient still needs to learn to live with fewer calories and more exercise after surgery.

Exercise does not have to be strenuous or painful, it can be as simple as a 30-minute walk. There are about as many exercise options as there are diets. The key is to find one that you enjoy, and to stick with it. Even small changes can make a difference: parking farther away at the grocery store, taking the stairs instead of the elevator, walking to the store instead of driving. If you incorporate 30 minutes of additional movement into your day, that will go a long way towards helping you shed pounds of unwanted fat.

Shedding unwanted fat is the key. Starving yourself is not the way to lose weight; you will lose muscle, which will slow down your metabolism. The more muscle mass you have, the higher your metabolism. What you want to lose is fat. You need to eat a balanced and nutritional diet. You need protein. You need carbohydrates (they are not BAD). You even need fats in your diet—just concentrate on the healthy ones.

Consuming fewer calories is difficult, especially in America where the motto is Super-Size everything. Stopping at just one serving or having smaller servings is not commonplace for most Americans. Most people do not take the time to eat slowly and savor the flavors of their food, therefore not allowing their brains and body to signal that they are getting full. Dr. Alan Hirsch, Director of the Smell and Taste Treatment and Research Foundation of Chicago, recognized that allowing for the sensory aspects of eating to be heightened would entice people to eat less. He invented Sensa, a safe and extremely effective weight loss program. Sensa works naturally and effectively by enhancing the smell and taste of foods that you eat—as perceived by the fullness center in your brain, which leads to eating less. Used properly, Sensa can result in safe and healthy weight loss. Self-control is a major factor in weight loss and Sensa helps by diminishing appetite.

Ultimately, the decision and commitment to lose weight needs to be owned by you. The tools you use to accomplish weight loss need to be tools that work effectively for you. There are numerous books and websites out there to help you with a proper diet. Try going to www.myhealthyweightandwellness. com for tips and advice from medical professionals.

The point here is that simply being overweight hurts your heart—so lose weight, and start now. In doing so, you will significantly decrease the chance of heart attacks and heart disease.

Appendix 1

Common Drugs Used in the Treatment of Heart Disease

M EDICATIONS ARE OFTEN PRESCRIBED to help prevent or control heart disease and reduce the risk of heart attack. Among the medications your doctor may prescribe are:

ARBs • Angiotensin II is a chemical that causes blood vessels to tighten. Angiotensin II receptor blockers (ARBs) are medications that block this powerful chemical thereby allowing blood vessels to relax. ARBs are used to treat high blood pressure, to prevent and treat heart failure, and to prevent kidney damage due to diabetes.

ASPIRIN • Aspirin helps to lower the risk of a heart attack for patients who have already experienced one. You should not take aspirin without the approval of your doctor.

DIGITALIS • Digitalis is prescribed to strengthen the pumping action of the heart. Digitalis helps the heart to contract harder, and also helps to slow the heart's rhythm in some patients.

ACE (ANGIOTENSIN CONVERTING ENZYME) INHIBITOR
• ACE drugs are often prescribed after a heart attack. ACE drugs help to control blood pressure and regulate a chemical that makes blood vessels become narrow.

BETA BLOCKER • Beta blockers are prescribed to reduce high blood pressure. They are also prescribed for chest pain. Beta blockers slow the heart and make it beat with less contracting force.

NITRATES (INCLUDING NITROGLYCERINE) • Nitrates are prescribed to relive angina. They relax blood vessels and help to stop chest pain.

CALCIUM CHANNEL BLOCKER • These drugs are also used to reduce high blood pressure as they relax blood vessels. They also relieve chest pain.

DIURETICS • Also called "water pills," diuretics decrease the amount of fluid in the body which helps the heart to function better.

BLOOD CHOLESTEROL-LOWERING AGENTS • "Statin" drugs are sometimes prescribed for patients with high cholesterol. These drugs lower the levels of "bad" (LDL) cholesterol levels in the blood.

THROMBOLYTIC AGENTS • These drugs thin the blood and are often given during a heart attack to break up a blood clot in a coronary artery in order to restore blood flow to the heart.

Warning. It is important to remember that all drugs have side effects. Even aspirin can be harmful if taken irresponsibly. Ask your doctor about the side effects of the medication you are taking, and if you experience any of them, contact your doctor immediately. Do not attempt to change or suddenly reduce the amount of medication you are taking without consulting your doctor. Doing so can have serious consequences.

Heart Healthy Recipes

Soups and Salads

Black Bean Soup
8 cups

1/2 cup diced celery
1/2 cup diced onion
2 tablespoons crushed fresh garlic
nonstick cooking spray
3 cups dried black beans (rinsed and sorted)
1 teaspoon celery salt
1 teaspoon chili powder
1/2 teaspoon ground red pepper
1/2 cup dry white wine
2 teaspoons Tabasco sauce

1. Over medium-low heat, saute the celery, onion, and garlic for about 10 minutes (or until the vegetables become translucent) in a nonstick skillet sprayed with

nonstick cooking spray. Pour the beans, celery salt, chili powder, red pepper, wine, and Tabasco sauce in a large pot.

2. Add the sauteed celery, onions, and garlic to the pot along with 12 cups of water. Over high heat, heat to boiling. Cover the pot, reduce heat to low, and cook for about 3 hours.

Per Serving
Calories: 110
Protein: 6 grams
Carbohydrates: 18 grams
Fat: 1 gram
Sodium: 19 milligrams

Potato Carrot Soup
10 Servings

6 white potatoes, peeled and diced (about 7 cups)
2 cups carrots, peeled and diced
2 cups diced onions
1/2 teaspoon celery seeds
1/2 teaspoon dried marjoram
2 1/2 cups skim milk
1 teaspoon freshly ground black pepper
1/2 teaspoon crushed red pepper flakes

1. In a large pot, bring 6 cups of water to a boil. Add the potatoes, carrots, onions, celery seeds, and marjoram, and cook, covered, for about 20 minutes or until the vegetables are very soft. Drain the vegetables, careful to reserve about 4 cups of the liquid (this will be used as stock water later).
2. Put the vegetables in a food processor and mix until smooth.
3. Pour the milk and 3 cups of the reserved stock into a pot and bring to a boil. Add the vegetables along with the black pepper and crushed red pepper. Cook for about 5 minutes. Add more stock for a thinner soup.

Per Serving
Calories: 155
Protein: 6 grams
Carbohydrates: 33 grams
Fat: less than 1 gram
Sodium: 46 milligrams

Macaroni Salad
4 servings

3 cups cooked elbow macaroni
1/2 cup diced celery
1/2 cup diced dill pickle
3 tablespoons diced pimento
2 tablespoons diced onion
3 tablespoons nonfat plain yogurt
1 teaspoon chopped fresh dill
1/2 teaspoon ground red pepper

4. In a large bowl, mix the pasta, celery, pickle, pimento, and onion.
5. In a separate bowl, blend together the yogurt, dill, and pepper.
6. Add the dressing to the pasta and mix thoroughly. Chill in the refrigerator for about 3 hours, to allow flavors to develop before serving.

Per Serving
Calories: 150
Protein: 5 grams
Carbohydrates: 30 grams
Fat: 1 gram
Sodium: 77 milligrams

Classic Potato Salad
4 servings

3 cups of white potatoes, peeled, cooked, and
    cut into 1-inch cubes
1/2 cup chopped celery
1/2 cup sweet pickle relish
1/2 cup sliced scallions (green onions)
1 tablespoon balsamic vinegar
1 tablespoon finely chopped fresh dill
1 1/2 teaspoons Dijon mustard
1/2 teaspoon ground white pepper

In a large bowl, combine all the ingredients, mixing well. Chill
in the refrigerator for at least 2 hours to allow flavors to develop
before serving.

Per Serving
Calories: 180
Protein: 4 grams
Carbohydrates: 43 grams
Fat: less than 1 gram
Sodium: 199 milligrams

Cole Slaw
4 servings

2 cups shredded green cabbage
2 cups shredded red cabbage
1/2 cup shredded carrots
1/2 cup diced onion
1/2 cup diced sweet pickles
3 tablespoons nonfat plain yogurt
2 tablespoons sugar
2 tablespoons freshly squeezed lemon juice
1/2 teaspoon lemon zest (grated from the lemon peel)

1. Mix all the ingredients thoroughly in a large bowl.
2. Chill in the refrigerator for 2 to 3 hours before serving.

Per Serving
Calories: 80
Protein: 2 grams
Carbohydrates: 20 grams
Fat: less than 1 gram
Sodium: 149 milligrams

String Bean Salad
6 servings

1 pound fresh string beans, steamed to desired tenderness
1/2 cup diced tomato
1/2 cup diced cucumber
1/2 cup diced green bell peppers
1/2 cup diced onion
3 tablespoons Dijon mustard
1 tablespoon balsamic vinegar

1. In a large bowl, combine the string beans, tomato, cucumber, bell peppers, and onion.
2. In a cup combine the mustard and vinegar. Pour the dressing over the vegetables and mix well.
3. Chill in the refrigerator for 1 to 2 hours to allow flavors to develop before serving.

Per Serving
Calories: 45
Protein: 2 grams
Carbohydrates: 9 grams
Fat: 1 gram
Sodium: 124 milligrams

Cucumber Salad
4 servings

2 1/2 cups thinly sliced unpeeled cucumbers
1/2 cup cubed tomatoes
1 tablespoon chopped fresh Italian parsley
1 teaspoon chopped fresh tarragon
1/2 cup diced onion
2 tablespoons balsamic vinegar
1 teaspoon freshly ground black pepper

1. Combine the cucumbers, tomatoes, parsley, tarragon, and onion in a large bowl.
2. In a cup, combine the vinegar and pepper and pour over the salad.
3. Mix well and chill in the refrigerator for about 3 hours to allow flavors to develop before serving.

Per Serving
Calories: 25
Protein: 1 gram
Carbohydrates: 5 grams
Fat: less than 1 gram
Sodium: 5 milligrams

Main Dishes

Codfish Cakes
8 Servings

1 pound cod fillets, steamed
1 teaspoon lemon juice
1 cup mashed potatoes
2 cloves garlic, minced
1 tablespoon finely minced rosemary leaves
3 teaspoons olive oil
1 teaspoon salt
1 teaspoon lemon pepper
1/2 teaspoon dry mustard
2 tablespoons bread crumbs
2 tablespoons flour

1. Put steamed fish into a large mixing bowl, sprinkle on lemon juice and toss. Add potatoes and gently fold into the dish.
2. In a small saucepan, saute garlic and rosemary in 1 teaspoon oil over medium heat for 1 minute, until garlic is lightly browned. Add garlic mixture, salt, lemon pepper, and mustard to the fish mixture and knead with your hands to mix thoroughly.
3. Shape into eight patties, and dredge in a combined mixture of bread crumbs and flour. Let chill in refrigerator for 1/2 hour.
4. In a large nonstick skillet, heat 1 teaspoon oil over medium-high heat. When hot, add four patties and cook for 3 minutes on each side, until well browned. Remove and drain on paper towels. Repeat with the remaining oil and patties.

Per Serving
Calories: 107
Carbohydrate: 8 grams
Fat: 3 grams
Sodium: 400 milligrams

Salmon Croquettes
8 servings

3 cloves garlic, minced
3 teaspoons olive oil
1 pound salmon fillet
1/2 cup dry vermouth
2 teaspoons butter
1 tablespoon flour
1/2 cup evaporated skim milk
1/2 cup mashed potatoes
1 teaspoon salt
2 teaspoons lemon pepper
2 tablespoons chopped parsley
2 tablespoons chopped chives
1 tablespoon chopped dill
1 egg, beaten
2 teaspoons lemon juice
1/2 cup flour
2 tablespoons bread crumbs

1. Sauté garlic in 1 teaspoon oil and set aside. 2. Steam salmon in vermouth for 10 minutes, until firm. Set aside to cool, and flake.
2. In a large saucepan, melt butter. When butter begins to bubble, stir in the tablespoon flour. Slowly add the

milk, stirring while pouring, until mixture is smooth and thickened. Add salmon, garlic, potatoes, salt, lemon pepper, parsley, chives, dill, egg, and lemon juice.

3. On a plate, combine 1/2 cup flour and bread crumbs. Run hands under cold water and shape salmon into eight patties and dredge in flour mixture. Chill for at least 1/2 hour.

4. In a nonstick skillet or cast-iron skillet, heat 1 teaspoon oil. Place four patties in the pan and cook 3 minutes on each side, until well browned. Drain on paper towels. Add remaining oil to the pan and cook the remaining four patties.

Per Serving
Calories: 129
Carbohydrates: 11 grams
Fat: 4 grams
Sodium: 379 milligrams

Skinless Fried Chicken
6 servings

6 skinless, bone-in chicken breast halves
2 cups 1 percent fat buttermilk
1/2 teaspoon salt
1 teaspoon freshly ground pepper
1 tablespoon lemon juice
1 teaspoon seasoned salt
2 teaspoons ground sage
2 teaspoons paprika
1/2 cup finely ground cracker crumbs

1 teaspoon baking powder
1/2 cup olive oil
1 cup flour

1. Split each halved chicken breast in half again. Soak each chicken piece in the buttermilk for 1 hour. Remove chicken from buttermilk mixture and pat dry. Discard milk.
2. Place chicken on a plate and sprinkle with salt, pepper, and lemon juice. Toss to mix evenly. In a paper bag, combine the seasoned salt, sage, paprika, cracker crumbs, flour and baking powder; shake the bag to mix.
3. In a large cast-iron or nonstick skillet, heat the oil over medium-high heat. Dredge chicken in the flour mixture and shake off excess. When oil is very hot, lay the chicken pieces in the pan, fleshy side down, and immediately reduce heat to medium. Cook for 10-12 minutes and turn the chicken over to cook for another 8-10 minutes, until chicken is golden brown. Remove and drain on paper towels.

Per Serving
Calories: 308
Carbohydrates: 25 grams
Fat: 7 grams
Sodium: 487 milligrams

Grilled Barbecued Chicken

6 Servings

6 boneless, skinless chicken breast halves
1/2 teaspoon salt
1/2 teaspoon freshly ground pepper
1 cup barbecue sauce

1. Put chicken in a shallow dish and sprinkle with salt and pepper. Pour on barbecue sauce, toss well, and let sit in refrigerator for at least 2 hours. Discard sauce or use as a baste for immediate use only.
2. Preheat grill for 15 minutes. Put chicken pieces, fleshy side down, on the hot grill and cook for 10 minutes, until chicken is slightly charred. Turn over and cook for 10 minutes more, basting occasionally.

Per Serving
Calories: 204
Carbohydrates: 14 grams
Fat: 3 grams
Sodium: 421 milligrams

Stuffed Pork Tenderloin with Vegetables
4 to 6 Servings

1/2 cup diced broccoli stems
1/2 cup diced cauliflower florets
1/2 cup diced carrots
1 egg white, lightly beaten
1 tablespoon fresh lime juice, plus 1 teaspoon
1/2 teaspoon dried rubbed sage
2 lean pork tenderloins (about 2 pounds)
2 tablespoons minced fresh garlic
1 teaspoon freshly ground black pepper nonstick cooking spray

1. Preheat oven to 400 F. In a bowl, mix the broccoli, cauliflower, carrots, egg white, tablespoon of lime juice, and sage. Set aside.
2. Along the length of each tenderloin, slice a pocket deep enough for half of the stuffing. Stuff each tenderloin with the stuffing, season them with garlic and pepper, and place them in a roasting pan lightly coated with cooking spray. Sprinkle additional lime juice on top of the tenderloins and spray each with cooking spray.
3. Cover the pan tightly with foil and roast for about 1 hour, turning the tenderloins halfway through cooking.

Per Serving
Calories: 215
Protein: 35 grams
Carbohydrates: 3 grams
Fat: 6 grams
Sodium: 121 milligrams

SIDE DISHES

Mississippi Dirty Rice
4 Servings

1 cup brown rice
1/2 cup ground all-white turkey
1/2 cup diced onion
2 tablespoons diced green bell pepper
1 tablespoon Soul Food Seasoning (under section entitled
    "Extras")
1 teaspoon chopped fresh garlic
1 teaspoon freshly ground black pepper
nonstick cooking spray

1. Bring 3 cups of water to a boil in a medium saucepan
    and add the rice. Cover and cook for about 50 min-
    utes over a low-medium heat; set aside.
2. Sauté the ground turkey, onion, green pepper, Soul
    Food Seasoning, garlic, and black pepper in a nonstick
    skillet lightly coated with nonstick cooking spray for
    about 15 minutes over a low heat.
3. In a large bowl, stir together the rice and turkey mix-
    ture.

Per Serving
Calories: 160
Protein: 9 grams
Carbohydrates: 26 grams
Fat: 2 grams
Sodium: 26 milligrams

Macaroni and Cheese
6 Servings

2 cups elbow macaroni
1/2 cup grated reduced-fat cheddar cheese
1/3 cup skim milk
2 tablespoons sliced scallions
1 egg white, lightly beaten
1 tablespoons nonfat Parmesan cheese topping

1. Cook the macaroni according to package instructions, and drain.
2. Place the macaroni in a large bowl and add the cheddar cheese, milk, scallions, and egg white. Stir well.
3. Preheat oven to 375 F. Place the macaroni in a non-stick casserole pan and sprinkle the Parmesan cheese on top. Bake about 25 minutes or until the top is browned and firm.

Per Serving
Calories: 155
Protein: 9 grams
Carbohydrates: 27 grams
Fat: less than 1 gram
Sodium: 115 milligrams

Baked Cheese Grits
4 Servings

1 cup uncooked grits
1/2 teaspoon reduced-fat margarine
3 egg whites, lightly beaten
1/2 cup grated reduced-fat cheddar cheese
1 teaspoon finely minced garlic

1. Preheat oven to 350 F. Bring 4 cups of water to a boil in a medium saucepan over high heat. Stir in the grits and reduce heat, cooking until they become thick, about 10 minutes.
2. Stir in the margarine, egg whites, cheese, and garlic, mixing thoroughly. Pour the mixture into a 9-inch nonstick pie pan and bake 40 to 50 minutes, or until lightly browned on the top. Remove from oven and cool in pan on wire rack. When grits cool, cut into small squares.

Per Serving
Calories: 75
Protein: 6 grams
Carbohydrates: 9 grams
Fat: 2 grams
Sodium: 234 milligrams

Unfried Hush Puppies
Makes 18 Hush Puppies

Nonstick cooking spray
1 1/2 cups yellow cornmeal
1/2 cup self-rising flour
2 1/2 teaspoons baking powder
1 tablespoon sugar
1/2 teaspoon salt
1/2 cup chopped onion
2 tablespoons chopped fresh parsley
2 cups skim milk
1 egg white, lightly beaten
1/2 cup water

Preheat oven to 400 F. Lightly coat an 18-cup muffin pan with nonstick cooking spray. Mix the cornmeal, flour, baking powder, sugar, and salt together. Fold in the onion, parsley, milk, egg white, and water. Pour the batter into the prepared muffin pan, filling each 1/2 full. Bake 20-25 minutes or until golden brown.

Per Serving
Calories: 60
Protein: 2 grams
Carbohydrates: 12 grams
Fat: less than 1 gram
Sodium: 272 milligrams

Jalapeno Corn Bread
6 Servings

nonstick cooking spray
2 cups yellow cornmeal
1 cup all-purpose flour
2 1/2 teaspoons baking powder
1 tablespoon sugar
2 diced fresh jalapeno peppers, seeded and chopped
1 cup skim milk
6 egg whites
1/2 cup cider vinegar

1. Preheat oven to 375 F. Lightly coat a 9 1/2 x 9 1/2-inch baking pan or 12-cup muffin pan with nonstick cooking spray. Mix the cornmeal, flour, baking powder, and sugar together in a large bowl. Add the peppers, milk, egg whites, and vinegar. Stir with a spoon until thoroughly mixed.
2. Spoon the batter into the prepared pan. Bake 45 to 50 minutes or until the top of the corn bread is firm and light brown. Cool in pan on wire rack.

Per Serving
Calories: 200
Protein: 8 grams
Carbohydrates: 39 grams
Fat: 1 gram
Sodium: 130 milligrams

Sweet Potato Biscuits
Makes about 14

Nonstick cooking spray
2 cups all-purpose flour
2 teaspoons baking powder
1 tablespoon granulated sugar
1/2 teaspoon salt
1 tablespoon reduced-fat margarine
1 cup mashed sweet potato
1/2 teaspoon ground cinnamon
1/2 teaspoon grated nutmeg
1 cup skim milk
1 egg white

1. Preheat oven to 400 F. Lightly coat a baking sheet with nonstick cooking spray. Using an electric mixer, combine the flour, baking powder, sugar, salt, and margarine. Then slowly mix in the sweet potatoes, cinnamon, nutmeg, and milk. Stir in the egg white.
2. On a lightly floured board, roll the dough out to 1/2 -inch thickness. Using a biscuit cutter, cut the dough into 2-inch circles and place them on the baking sheet. Bake about 25 minutes or until they are firm in the center.

Per Serving
Calories: 100
Protein: 3 grams
Carbohydrates: 20 grams
Fat: less than 1 gram
Sodium: 290 milligrams

Mashed Potatoes
8 servings

8 large potatoes, scrubbed
1 tablespoon butter
2 tablespoons minced chives
1/2 cup 1 percent fat buttermilk, warmed
2 tablespoons reduced-fat mayonnaise
1 teaspoon salt
Freshly ground white pepper

1. Boil potatoes in water to cover for 20 to 25 minutes, or until tender when a fork is inserted. When fairly cool, drain and grate, or put through a potato ricer, including the skins, into a large bowl.
2. Add butter and chives, and mash. With a large fork, whip the potatoes while adding buttermilk. Add mayonnaise, salt, and pepper, and whip again.

Per Serving
Calories: 119
Carbohydrates: 21 grams
Fat: 2 grams
Sodium: 306 milligrams

VEGETABLES

String Beans with Potatoes
8 servings

1 tablespoon olive oil

1 whole onion

1 pound green beans, trimmed

1 pound red new potatoes, quartered

1 teaspoon salt

1/2 teaspoon grated lemon zest

1 tablespoon lemon juice

1/2 teaspoon freshly ground white pepper

1. Heat olive oil in large heavy skillet. Sauté onion in oil for 15 minutes, until golden.
2. Blanch beans for 5 minutes in boiling water, then plunge into a bowl of ice water. Drain.
3. Add beans to the onion mixture in the skillet, and add potatoes, salt, and lemon zest. Cook over medium heat for 30 minutes, or until potatoes are soft. Add lemon juice and pepper.

Per Serving

Calories: 81

Carbohydrates: 15 grams

Fat: 1 gram

Sodium: 342 milligrams

Vegetables

String Beans with Potatoes
8 servings

1 tablespoon olive oil
1 whole onion
1 pound green beans, trimmed
1 pound red new potatoes, quartered
1 teaspoon salt
1/2 teaspoon grated lemon zest
1 tablespoon lemon juice
1/2 teaspoon freshly ground white pepper

1. Heat olive oil in large heavy skillet. Sauté onion in oil for 15 minutes, until golden.
2. Blanch beans for 5 minutes in boiling water, then plunge into a bowl of ice water. Drain.
3. Add beans to the onion mixture in the skillet, and add potatoes, salt, and lemon zest. Cook over medium heat for 30 minutes, or until potatoes are soft. Add lemon juice and pepper.

Per Serving
Calories: 81
Carbohydrates: 15 grams
Fat: 1 gram
Sodium: 342 milligrams

Fried Green Tomatoes
4 servings

6 large green tomatoes (about 3 pounds)
2 tablespoons lemon juice
1/2 cup cornmeal
2 teaspoons freshly ground black pepper
nonstick cooking spray

1. Slice each tomato into 1/2 -inch-thick slices. Sprinkle the lemon juice on the tomatoes.
2. Mix the cornmeal and black pepper in a plastic bag. Put the tomato slices into the bag and shake well.
3. Coat a cast-iron skillet or nonstick sauté pan with nonstick cooking spray. Fry the tomatoes, over medium-high heat, until they are light brown on each side.

Per Serving
Calories: 105
Protein: 3 grams
Carbohydrates: 22 grams
Fat: 2 grams
Sodium: 22 milligrams

Black-Eyed Peas
8–10 Servings

3 cups dried black-eyed peas

1 cup chopped skinless smoked turkey breast

1 cup chopped onion

1/2 cup chopped carrot

1/2 cup chopped celery

2 tablespoons cider vinegar

2 tablespoons Soul Food Seasoning (under section entitled "Extras")

1 teaspoon fresh ground black pepper

1. Rinse and sort the peas. Place them in a large pot with enough water to cover and bring to boil. Once boiling, remove the pot from the heat, cover, and let stand for 1- 1/2 hours.

2. Add the remaining ingredients and additional water if necessary to cover the peas. Place a lid on the pot, and cook on a low-medium heat for 1 hour, or until the peas are tender. Make sure there is enough water added in the pot to cover the peas throughout the cooking time.

Per Serving

Calories: 95

Protein: 9 grams

Carbohydrates: 14 grams

Fat: less than 1 gram

Sodium: 28 milligrams

Collard Greens
8 Servings

3 pounds collard greens, rinsed and chopped
1/2 pound smoked turkey breast, cubed
1 cup nonfat chicken broth
1/2 cup minced onion
1 teaspoon crushed red pepper flakes
1 teaspoon minced celery
1 teaspoon freshly ground black pepper

1. Place the collard greens and turkey breast in a large pot. Cover them with water, and cook on a medium heat, covered, for 20 minutes.
2. Add the chicken broth, onion, red pepper flakes, celery, and black pepper, and cook on a low-medium heat, covered, for about 45 minutes.

Per Serving
Calories: 95
Protein: 11 grams
Carbohydrates: 13 grams
Fat: 1 gram
Sodium: 78 milligrams

Desserts

Deep-Dish Apple Pie
8 servings

10 large tart apples
Juice of 1 lemon
1/2 cup sugar
2 tablespoons pie spice (see recipe in this section)
1/2 teaspoon grated lemon zest
1 teaspoon finely chopped crystallized ginger
2 tablespoons ground tapioca
3 teaspoons butter
1 9-inch piecrust (see next page)
Milk

1. Preheat the oven to 325 degrees F. Butter a 9-inch deep-dish pie plate and set aside. Peel, core, and quarter the apples. Slice the apples 1/8 inch thick and place them in a large bowl of water mixed with the lemon juice.
2. In a small bowl, combine the sugar, pie spice, zest, ginger, and tapioca. Divide into three parts. Drain the apples and divide into thirds.
3. Place the first layer of apples in the baking dish, overlapping the apples if necessary. Sprinkle one third of the spice mixture evenly over the apples and top with 1 teaspoon butter. Repeat with a second and third layer.
4. Cover with the piecrust dough. Crimp the edges with a fork dipped in milk, and cut three slits in the top. Bake for 40 minutes, until golden brown on top. Let come to room temperature before slicing.

Per Serving
Calories: 289
Carbohydrates: 55 grams
Fat: 8 grams
Sodium: 159 milligrams

9-Inch Piecrust

1 cup all-purpose unbleached flour
1/2 teaspoon salt
1 teaspoon sugar
1/2 cup sweet butter, chilled
3 tablespoons nonfat sour cream, or 1 percent fat buttermilk,
    chilled
1 teaspoon ice water

1. Sift the flour, salt, and sugar into a large mixing bowl. Cut the butter into small chunks and, using your fingers, briskly rub the butter into the flour. (This step requires a bit of speed; otherwise, you'll end up with an oily crust.)
2. When the mixture resembles coarse meal, add the sour cream. Using a fork, work the sour cream into the meal. Add ice water and pull the mixture together to form a ball. Knead the dough lightly two to three times. Reshape the dough into a ball again, wrap in plastic, and refrigerate for at least 1 hour.
3. Turn the ball out onto a lightly floured surface and roll out to the desired diameter (9 inches).

Note: For a prebaked pie shell, preheat the oven to 375 degrees F. Prick the crust with a fork and bake for 10 to 12 minutes, until golden. Cool.

Per Serving
Calories: 105
Carbohydrates: 12 grams
Fat: 5 grams
Sodium: 139 milligrams

Lemon Pound Cake
12 servings

1 cup sugar
1 cup unsweetened applesauce
4 egg whites, at room temperature
2 tablespoons lemon extract
3 cups all-purpose flour
1/2 cup skim milk
1 1/2 teaspoons baking powder
2 teaspoons lemon zest
1/2 cup all-natural lemon preserves (no sugar added)
nonstick cooking spray

1. Preheat oven to 350 degrees F. With an electric mixer, beat the sugar and applesauce. Mix in the egg whites and lemon extract. Add the flour and milk alternately, using the flour first and last. Mix in the baking powder.
2. Pour the cake batter into a 10-inch tube pan (or one sprayed with cooking spray) and bake about 1 1/2 hours. Remove the cake from the pan and let it cool for about 20 minutes. Heat the 1/2 cup of lemon preserves in a saucepan for about 1 minute (until melted enough to pour) and drizzle over the cake.

Per Serving
Calories: 215
Protein: 4 grams
Carbohydrates: 29 grams
Fat: less than 1 gram
Sodium: 56 milligrams

Banana Pudding
8 servings

1/2 cup sugar
2 tablespoons cornstarch
2 cups evaporated skim milk
2 teaspoons vanilla extract
2 1/2 cups vanilla wafer crumbs
3 cups bananas, sliced
3 large egg whites, at room temperature
ground cinnamon

1. Preheat oven to 400 degrees F. Combine the sugar, cornstarch, and milk in a medium saucepan. Cook over a low heat, stirring constantly until the mixture thickens like pudding. Add the vanilla extract.
2. In a 9-inch or 10-inch casserole dish, arrange a layer of vanilla wafers (touching each other). Arrange a layer of banana slices on top of the wafers. Repeat with wafers and bananas.
3. Pour the thickened pudding mixture over the bananas. Using an electric mixer, beat the egg whites until stiff, then spread on top of the pudding. Sprinkle cinnamon on top.
4. Bake the pudding until the surface of the egg whites begins to brown. Let the custard cool for about 2 hours

before serving.

Per Serving
Calories: 200
Protein: 7 Grams
Carbohydrates: 35 grams
Fat: 4 grams
Sodium: 129 milligrams

About the Authors

Hilton M. Hudson II, M.D., F.A.C.S. is the Chief of Cardiotho-racic Surgery, and a practicing heart surgeon at Franciscan Physicians Hospital, President & CEO of Hilton Publishing Company, and Chairman of the Board of the Health Literacy Foundation. He graduated cum laude from Wabash College, and received his medical training at Indiana University School of Medicine. He trained in general surgery at Boston City Hospital and Boston University Hospital, and completed his car- diothoracic training at Ohio State University. Dr. Hudson is certi- fied in thoracic cardiac surgery. He is a diplomat of the American Board of Thoracic Surgery, a Fellow of the American College of Surgeons, a member of the Association of African American Cardiovascular Surgeons, and a Fellow of the College of Chest Physicians. He belongs to the American Medical Association, the National Medical Association, Boston Surgical Society, the Association of Black Cardiologists, the Hinton-Wright Society at Harvard Medical School, and the Zollinger Surgical Society. He lives in Chicago, Illinois.

Karol E. Watson, M.D., Ph.D., F.A.C.C. is Associate Professor of Medicine and Cardiology at the David Geffen School of Medicine at UCLA. She is also Director of the UCLA Women's Cardiovascular Center and Co-Director of the UCLA Program in Preventive Cardiology. Dr. Watson is a graduate of Stanford University and Harvard Medical School, where she graduated magna cum laude. She completed her residency in Internal Medicine and fellowship in Cardiology at UCLA where she also received her Ph.D. in Physiology. Dr. Watson is a founding board member of the National Lipid Association, a member and former officer of the Association of Black Cardiologists, and a fellow of the American Heart Association (AHA) and the American College of Cardiology (ACC). She has received numerous awards and honors and was named one of "America's Top Physicians" by *Black Enterprise* magazine and one of Los Angeles' "Super Doctors" by *Tu Ciudad* magazine. Dr. Watson lives in Los Angeles, California.

Richard Allen Williams, M.D. is Clinical Professor of Medicine at the David Geffen School of Medicine at the University of California Los Angeles (UCLA), is the Founder of the Association of Black Cardiologists, and is President & CEO of the Minority Health Institute. He was head of the Cardiology Section of the West Los Angeles VA Hospital for several years. He graduated with honors from Harvard University, received his medical degree from the State University of New York Downstate Medical Center, performed his internship at the University of California San Francisco Medical Center, his Internal Medicine residency at the Los Angeles County-USC Medical Center, and Cardiology fellowship at Harvard Medical School and Brigham and Women's Hospital in Boston, where he was also a faculty member.